T0257864

Advanced Topics in Arthroplasty

Advanced Topics in Arthroplasty

Edited by **Robert Berry**

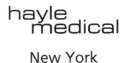

New York

Published by Hayle Medical,
30 West, 37th Street, Suite 612,
New York, NY 10018, USA
www.haylemedical.com

Advanced Topics in Arthroplasty
Edited by Robert Berry

International Standard Book Number: 978-1-63241-020-7 (Hardback)

This book contains information obtained from authentic and highly regarded sources. Copyright for all individual chapters remain with the respective authors as indicated. A wide variety of references are listed. Permission and sources are indicated; for detailed attributions, please refer to the permissions page. Reasonable efforts have been made to publish reliable data and information, but the authors, editors and publisher cannot assume any responsibility for the validity of all materials or the consequences of their use.

The publisher's policy is to use permanent paper from mills that operate a sustainable forestry policy. Furthermore, the publisher ensures that the text paper and cover boards used have met acceptable environmental accreditation standards.

Trademark Notice: Registered trademark of products or corporate names are used only for explanation and identification without intent to infringe.

Printed in the United States of America.

Contents

Preface

Over the recent decade, advancements and applications have progressed exponentially. This has led to the increased interest in this field and projects are being conducted to enhance knowledge. The main objective of this book is to present some of the critical challenges and provide insights into possible solutions. This book will answer the varied questions that arise in the field and also provide an increased scope for furthering studies.

Novel technologies, advancements in implant design and developments in surgical technique have better results after joint substitution and have led to a declined rate of difficulties. It is no surprise that the number of arthroplasties grows constantly every year; and nowadays, more than one million people go through the procedure annually worldwide. Focusing at dissemination of scientific research this book offers a thorough sketch of the current advancement of technology and surgical techniques in arthroplasty. Complications after arthroplasty, alternatives to arthroplasty and periprosthetic infections have been analytically examined by the contributing authors. This book is a valuable source of reference for students and practitioners.

I hope that this book, with its visionary approach, will be a valuable addition and will promote interest among readers. Each of the authors has provided their extraordinary competence in their specific fields by providing different perspectives as they come from diverse nations and regions. I thank them for their contributions.

Editor

Complications After Arthroplasty

Complications Following Total Hip Arthroplasty

Asim Rajpura and Tim Board

Additional information is available at the end of the chapter

1. Introduction

Total hip arthroplasty (THA) is an increasingly common and successful operation, with 76,759 procedures logged in the National Joint Registry for England and Wales in 2010 [1]. Overall satisfaction rates rank amongst the highest of any joint replacement procedure, with over 90% reporting a good to excellent overall outcome [2, 3].

Complications related to THA can be classified as either procedure specific or systemic. Advances in technology, anaesthesiology and surgical technique have resulted in an overall temporal decrease in complication rates despite the increasing incidence of co-morbidities in the patient population [4]. Table 1 highlights rates of complications most commonly encountered after THA.

2. Systemic / non-surgical

2.1. Thromboembolic complications

Deep Vein Thrombosis

Distal deep vein thrombosis (DVT) can range from being asymptomatic, to resulting in long term valvular damage resulting in chronic venous insufficiency. Proximal propagation can result in more serious pulmonary embolism. The overall incidence of DVT, including both radiologically diagnosed asymptomatic DVT and symptomatic DVT, post THA in early studies was reported to be as high as 70% without any form of prophylaxis [15]. Recent systematic review of several randomised control trials concerned with DVT prophylaxis has estimated this figure to be around 44% [16]. The recent FOTO study has shown a symptomatic DVT rate of 1.3% in THA patients with extended duration [36 day) chemical prophylaxis [8].

The overall combined incidence of asymptomatic and symptomatic DVT with prophylaxis has not declined with time, converse to the findings with knee arthroplasty in which the incidence has declined significantly [17]. This may be due to the increasing frequency of co morbidities within patients undergoing THA which act as risk factors for DVT.

Systemic		Procedure Specific	
Complication	Rate	Complication	Rate
Subclinical Fat Embolism	90%[5]	Dislocation (Posterior approach with repair)	0.49%[6]
Symptomatic Fat Embolism	Unknown	Leg length discrepancy (patient perceived)	30%[7]
Symptomatic Deep Vein Thrombosis with prophylaxis	1.3%[8]	Infection	1.08%[9]
Symptomatic Pulmonary Embolism with prophylaxis	0.5 – 0.6%[10]	Aseptic Loosening	2% failure rate at 15 years (Corail uncemented stem) [11] 3.2% failure rate at 30 years (Exeter Cemented Stem)[12]
Mortality	0.29 – 0.6%[4]	Periprosthetic Fracture (Postoperative femoral)	1.1%[13]
Myocardial Infarction	0.5%[10]	Heterotopic Ossification (Grade III/IV)	3 – 7%[14]

Table 1. Complication rates for Total Hip Arthroplasty

THA is thought to mainly affect 2 limbs of Virchow's triad, namely hypercoagulability and venous stasis. Activation of the coagulation cascade begins during surgery, primarily during preparation and insertion of the femoral prosthesis, with cemented prostheses providing a greater stimulus than uncemented implants [18]. Whether this increases the incidence of DVT with cemented fixation is unclear as the evidence is inconclusive [15, 19]. Venous haemodynamics are also altered not only during surgery, but also for up to 6 weeks post operatively [20]. Significant reductions in venous capacitance and outflow are seen in both legs, with greater changes seen in the operated leg, and this has been shown to correlate directly with the incidence of postoperative DVT [20]. Complete femoral vein occlusion has also been noted during THA, particularly during the posterior approach when the limb is internally rotated and flexed for operation on the femur [18].

Numerous risk factors for postoperative DVT have been identified. Major risk factors in approximate order of importance include: hip fracture, malignancy, antiphospholipid syndrome, immobility, previous history of DVT, use of selective oestrogen receptor modulators, oral contraceptives, morbid obesity, stroke, atherosclerosis and a ASA greater than 3 [21]. However 50% of patients who develop DVT have no identifiable clinical risk factor [21]. Genetic predispositions include antithrombin III and protein C deficiency and prothrombin gene mutation [21]. In order to aid recognition of 'at risk' patients, the National Institute for Health and Clinical Excellence (NICE) has published a table of relevant patient related risk factors as shown in Table 2 [16].

Active cancer or cancer treatment	Active heart or respiratory failure
Acute medical illness	Age over 60 years
Antiphospholipid syndrome	Behcet's disease
Central venous catheter in situ	Continuous travel of more than 3hours approximately 4weeks before or after surgery
Immobility (for example, paralysis or limb in plaster)	Inflammatory bowel disease
Myeloproliferative diseases	Nephrotic syndrome
Obesity (body mass index > 30kg/m2]	Paraproteinaemia
Paroxysmal nocturnal haemoglobinuria	Personal or family history of VTE
Pregnancy or puerperium	Recent myocardial infarction or stroke
Severe infection	Use of oral contraceptives or hormonal replacement therapy
Varicose veins with associated phlebitis	
Inherited Thrombophilias for example:	
High levels of coagulation factors (for example, Factor VIII)	Hyperhomocysteinaemia
Low activated protein C resistance (for example, Factor V Protein C, S and antithrombin deficiencies Leiden)	
Prothrombin 2021A gene mutation	

Table 2. Patient related risk factors for Venous Thromboembolism [16]

Prophylaxis against DVT begins with the type of anaesthesia used. Regional compared to general anaesthesia has been shown to reduce the risk of DVT post THA by over 50% [22, 23]. This is thought to be due to the relative hyperkinetic blood flow seen in the lower limbs during regional anaesthesia compared to general anaesthesia, and the stabilising effect of local anaesthetics on the cell membranes of vascular endothelium and platelets [24]. Mechanical and chemical prophylaxis remains a somewhat contentious issue, with various differing opinions existing regarding prophylaxis regimes. Numerous randomised controlled trials exist supporting the use of mechanical methods such as pneumatic compression devices (figure 1) and chemical methods such as low molecular weight heparins and fondaparinux, a factor Xa inhibitor [25-34].

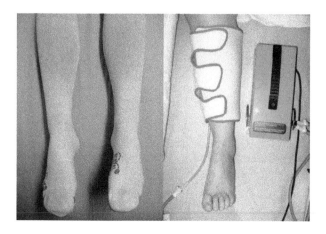

Figure 1. Left: Thrombo-Embolic Deterrent Stockings, Right: Flotron pumps (Huntleigh Healthcare Ltd, Luton, UK)

There has been recent increasing interest in oral factor Xa inhibitors such as Rivaroxaban and Apixaban. The RECORD trial has demonstrated greater effectiveness for oral Rivaroxaban compared to subcutaneous Enoxaparin with equal side effect profiles [35, 36]. Pooled analysis of the ADVANCE-2 and ADVANCE-3 trials has also demonstrated greater efficacy for oral Apixaban compared to subcutaneous Enoxaparin [37]. There has been some recent concern however regarding the increased rate of wound complications, specifically with the use of Rivaroxaban [38]. A retrospective analysis by Jensen et al. demonstrated a greater return to theatre rate for wound complications such as prolonged drainage and haematoma associated with the use of Rivaroxaban compared to Tinzaparin [38]. The authors suggest that trial data to date has not fully evaluated the complications profile of Rivaroxaban, as only major bleeding was used as a primary outcome measure, and further randomised trials are necessary to examine rates of surgical complications.

Current recommendations by National Institute for Health and Clinical Excellence (NICE) in England state that, THA patients should be offered mechanical prophylaxis in the form of intermittent pneumatic compression devices or compression stockings, and chemical prophylaxis with either low molecular weight heparin, Fondaparinux, Rivaroxaban or Dabigatran. This should be continued for 28-35 days post operatively [39].

2.2. Pulmonary embolism

DVTs that propagate proximally have the potential embolise to the lungs resulting in pulmonary emboli (PE). Mild emboli can be asymptomatic, whereas massive embolism can be fatal, and PE is one of the leading causes of mortality post THA. Rates for symptomatic pulmonary embolism in recent large case series of primary THA in which chemical prophylaxis was used, has been between 0.51-0.6% [10, 40]. In the absence of prophylaxis this is estimated to be around 3%, with approximately 6% of symptomatic PEs post THA result in fatality [16].

As with DVT, both mechanical and chemical methods such as pneumatic compression pumps and low molecular weight heparins have been shown to provide effective prophylaxis against symptomatic PE [25, 41-44]. However due to the low rate of fatal PE, trials and even meta-analyses have failed to demonstrate statistically significant effects on the rate of fatal PE by using thromboembolic prophylaxis [45]. Power analysis indicates a trial involving 67,000 patients would be needed to demonstrate a statistically significant difference [46].

Vena Caval filters as shown in figure 2 can also be used to prevent migration of venous emboli into the pulmonary circulation. However no RCTs exist supporting their use in surgical patients and significant complications such as pneumothorax, air embolism and arteriovenous fistulae can develop either during their placement or post procedure [47]. UK NICE guidelines therefore recommend their use in patients with recent or existing thromboembolic disease in whom anticoagulation is contraindicated [39].

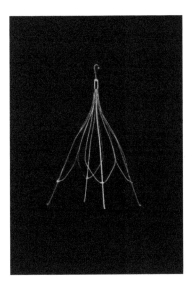

Figure 2. Retrievable Inferior Vena Caval Filter, courtesy of Cook Medical

2.3. Fat embolism

During insertion of the femoral component, rises in intramedullary pressure can force medullary fat and marrow contents into the venous circulation via the metaphyseal vessels [48-50]. Fat and marrow embolus can then pass into and through the pulmonary circulation depending on the size of the emboli [51, 52]. Large emboli can lodge within the pulmonary circulation leading to pulmonary hypertension and haemodynamic instability. Trans-pulmonary passage of micro-emboli can result in cerebral embolism potentially causing neurological complications [51, 53].

Subclinical fat embolisation can been detected in up to 90% of patients undergoing THA [5]. However the exact incidence of fat embolism syndrome characterised by the classic triad of respiratory insufficiency, neurolgic symptoms and upper body petechiae is unknown [54].

Measures to reduce the risk of fat embolism include medullary lavage to reduce the fat load during cement pressurisation [55]. Vacuum cementation techniques using drainage cannulae have also been shown to be effective in reducing the intramedullary pressure rises during cementation therefore reducing the risk of emboli [56]. Treatment of established fat embolism syndrome is essentially supportive, frequently requiring intensive care unit admission for respiratory support.

3. Mortality and cardiorespiratory complications

Published rates for mortality following primary THA are low, ranging from between 0.29% to 0.6% [4, 10]. Mortality rates have declined slightly with time despite the increasing incidence of relevant co-morbidities [4]. Cardiovascular complications account for the most common cause of death [57].

Age has been identified as one of the strongest predictors of post operative mortality after joint arthroplasty [10]. Octegenarians have been shown to have a mortality rate 3.4 times higher than patients between 65-79 years of age and were 2.4 times more likely to suffer a post operative myocardial infarction [58]. Other significant risk factors for post operative mortality and morbidity include male sex, smoking and higher American Society of Anesthesiologists' (ASA) grade which is representative of relevant significant co-morbidities such as artherosclerosis, diabetes, renal impairment and valvular disease [10, 59, 60]. Greenfield et al. found that the incidence of morbidity after THA varied from 3% to 41% when comparing those with the lowest and highest incidence of co-morbidities [61]. The role of anaesthesia is somewhat controversial. Some studies suggest regional compared to general anaesthesia may reduce the risk of thromboembolic and cardiorespiratory complications and short term mortality [62, 63]. Others have shown no difference between the 2 groups in terms of morbidity and mortality [64]. Therefore no conclusive evidence exists supporting one form of anaesthesia, but the overall consensus would appear to favour regional techniques [54].

4. Procedure specific / surgical complications

4.1. Dislocation

Dislocation is the 3rd most common cause for revision after THA [65]. Published rates for dislocation after primary THA vary widely between 0.2% to 7% [66]. Up to 70% of dislocations occur early within 6 weeks [67]. Early dislocation carries a better prognosis compared to late dislocation which is defined as occurring after 3 months, as late dislocation usually has a multifactiorial aetiology including component wear and soft tissue laxity [68, 69]. Approximately a third of dislocating THAs managed conservatively after the first episode will go on to become recurrent dislocators [67]. Risk factors for dislocation can be classified as either patient, surgery or implant related.

4.2. Patient related risk factors

Patients with neuromuscular and cognitive disorders such as cerebral palsy, muscular dystrophy and dementia, have been shown to have higher rates of dislocation [70]. Fracture as the primary indication for surgery is the indication most strongly linked with dislocation [71]. This is thought to be due to the lack of capsular hypertrophy normally seen with osteoarthritis which provides additional stability. Previous hip surgery of any sort has also been shown to double the risk of dislocation [68]. Factors such as height, weight, age and sex of the patient have not been conclusively shown to affect the rates of dislocation [67].

4.3. Surgical risk factors

Surgical factors include surgical approach, soft tissue tension, component design and orientation, and surgeon experience. The majority of dislocations occur in a posterior direction and therefore the posterior approach has been deemed to be the approach with the highest risk of dislocation. Early data supported this theory with Woo et al reporting a rate of 5.8% for posterior approach compared to 2.3% for an antero-lateral approach [68]. However recent research investigating the role of posterior capsular and external rotator repair has shown comparable rates to other approaches [72, 73]. A recent meta-analysis has shown a reduction of the dislocation rate from 4.46% to 0.49% by carrying out a posterior soft tissue repair [6]. Therefore with meticulous soft tissue repair, surgical approach should have little effect on dislocation rates. Besides the posterior structures, the glutei and joint capsule also provide soft tissue tension reducing dislocation risk. Therefore following a transtrochanteric approach, trochanteric non union greater than 1cm can result in abductor insufficiency increasing the rates of dislocation by over 6 fold [68]. Inadequate offset is another factor affecting soft tissue tension and has been shown to increase dislocation risk [74].

4.4. Implant related factors

Component positioning and design both play key roles in reducing dislocation risk. "Safe zones" for acetabular cup position are defined as an abduction angle of $40° ± 10°$ and anteversion of $20° ± 10°$ [75, 76]. With a posterior approach reduced cup anteversion has been shown to be a major risk factor for dislocation [77]. Archbold et al. have suggested the use of the transverse acetabular ligament as a landmark to judge cup anteversion [78]. Using this technique they reported a 0.6% dislocation rate using a posterior approach with soft tissue repair. How this relates to the traditionally defined safe zones is currently being examined. Femoral component positioning has been less well studied. Recent studies have suggested the use of a 'combined anteversion' technique in which the acetabular and stem combined anteversion should be $35° ± 10°$ [79, 80].

Femoral head size also affects stability. Larger heads provide more favourable head-neck ratios, reducing possible impingement, and seat deeper within the acetabulum requiring a greater 'jump distance' to cause dislocation as illustrated in figure 3. Such advantages have been validated using cadaveric and computer modelling [81-83]. Clinical data from both the Norwegian and Australian joint registries has also shown a reduction in rates of revision for dislocation with increasing head size [84, 85].

Surgeon experience is another factor that has been identified in influencing dislocation rates. Hedlundh et al. found that surgeons who had performed less than 30 THAs had a double rate of dislocation compared to more experienced surgeons [86]. A recent systematic review has also demonstrated reduced dislocation rates with increased surgical volume [87].

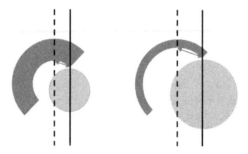

Figure 3. Jumping Distance highlighted by red arrow demonstrates distance the head needs to travel before dislocation occurs. Increasing head size increases this distance

5. Management

Management of dislocation initially involves closed reduction which is usually successful in the majority of cases. This should be performed ideally under anaesthesia with muscle relaxation to reduce the chance of damage to the femoral head [88, 89]. Some surgeons advocate the use of an abduction brace after reduction but little evidence exists supporting their use.

Indications for operative intervention include recurrent or irreducible dislocation, component malposition, soft tissue laxity and dislocation due to impingement. Strategies during revision include component realignment, removal of osteophytes causing impingement, modular component exchange to increase head size and improve head-neck ratio, liner exchange if worn and addressing soft tissue laxity using capsulorrhaphy, trochanteric advancement or tendon allografts.

Selected patients unsuitable for major revision surgery can be treated with posterior lip augmentation devices (PLAD) as shown in figure 4. These consist of a C shaped piece of UHMWPE and a steel backing plate, and are applied to the posterior lip of the acetabulum and held in place with up to 5 screws. This constrains the head within the augmented socket. Contraindications to its use include gross component malalignment and loosening. McConway et al. reviewed 307 recurrently dislocating THAs treated with PLADs [90]. Persistent instability occurred in only 5 patients [1.6%) and there was no evidence of accelerated loosening affecting the acetabular component.

Salvage procedures for failed revision or uncorrectable aetiology include the use of constrained cups or conversion to bipolar hemiarthroplasty. However both of these procedures are associated with poor functional outcome and constrained cups can result in premature loosening [70]. Therefore their use is usually reserved for low demand patients. The final salvage option is Girdlestone resection for the unreconstructable hip.

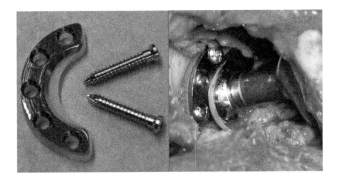

Figure 4. Posterior Lip Augementation Device (PLAD, Depuy, UK)

5.1. Leg length discrepancy

Leg length discrepancy (LLD) is the most common cause of patient dissatisfaction and subsequent litigation after THA [91]. LLD can result in nerve palsies, abnormal gait, lower back pain and reduced functional outcome [92]. Wylde et al. showed up to 30% of patients after primary THA can have a perceived LLD, but only 36% of these had an anatomic LLD greater than 5mm [7].

Nerve palsies are potentially the most serious complications of LLD. Sciatic and peroneal nerve palsies have both been associated with limb lengthening. Edwards et al suggested sciatic and peroneal nerve palsies are associated with lengthening greater than 4 and 3.8cm respectively [93]. Farrell et al however found an average lengthening of only 1.7cm was a significant risk factor for nerve palsies [94]. Therefore safe limits for limb lengthening before traction nerve palsies develop are yet to be defined, and it may be that any minor degree of lengthening may make the nerve more susceptible to other trauma [94].

Minor LLD less than 1cm is usually well tolerated by patients. However LLD greater than 2cm has been shown to significantly affect the gait cycle, increasing physiological demand [95]. LLD greater than 3cm in the elderly was shown to cause significant increases in heart rate and quadriceps activity in the lengthened limb, which may be especially relevant in patients with cardio-respiratory co-morbidities [95].

Avoiding potential problems with LLD begins with patient history and examination. It is crucial to determine patient perceived leg length in order to counsel the patient effectively regarding likely outcomes. True leg length can then be determined, measuring from the ipsilateral anterior superior iliac spine to the medial malleolus, followed by apparent leg length by measuring from the umbilicus to the medial malleolus. Apparent leg length can be affected by pelvic obliquity secondary to either lumbar spine pathology or contractures about the hip. Significant LLD due to fixed pelvic obliquity secondary to chronic lumbar spine pathology cannot usually be corrected as it may involve significant shortening or lengthening. With pelvic obliquity secondary to contractures, the true length only needs to be corrected as after the THA the pelvis will balance with time [96].

Radiographs can also be used to determine leg length by referencing the position of the lesser trochanter in relation to a line drawn across the inferior aspect of the pelvis as shown in figure 5. Templating can then be carried out to determine the correct level of the neck cut for the femoral prosthesis and the position of the acetabular component in order to determine the new hip centre. Both of these directly affect leg length.

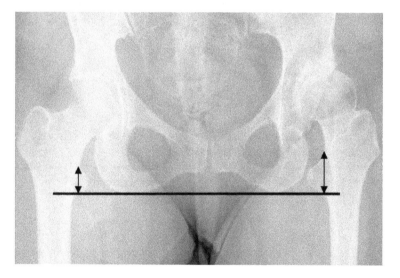

Figure 5. Radiographic estimation of LLD can be made by measuring vertically from the top of the lesser trochanter to a line drawn across the inferior margin of the pelvis

Intraoperative methods include the use of measurements taken from reference pins placed in the pelvis to a mark on the greater trochanter [97-99]. Mihalko et al described using a large fragment screw placed above the superior rim of the acetabulum and marking a point on the greater trochanter a fixed distance from this prior to dislocation. After insertion of the prostheses this distance was rechecked giving an indication of leg length changes [98]. Shiramizu et al used a similar method but with a steimann pin in the ilium and a custom calliper to measure the distances [99]. They found a mean LLD of only 2.1mm with this method.

Minor LLD postoperatively can be treated using a shoe raise. Prescription of such devices should be delayed for 3-6 months to allow any residual pelvic tilt secondary to contractures to resolve as the soft tissues can progressively relax. Failure of conservative measures and symptoms such as severe pain, nerve palsies and instability can necessitate surgical intervention. Shortening can be treated using soft tissue release and exchange of modular heads to give modest changes in leg length or more extensive surgery such as exchange of the femoral component to give greater neck length or offset. Lengthening can also be treated with component exchange but secondary procedures such as trochanteric advancement or the use of larger heads or stems with increased offset may be needed to maintain stability [100].

5.2. Infection

Infection post THA is potentially one of the most catastrophic and challenging to treat complications. During the early development of THA, Charnley reported a deep infection rate of 9.4% in unventilated operating theatres [101]. This initial unacceptably high deep infection rate stimulated the development of several prophylactic measures including ultraclean laminar air flow ventilation and peri-operative antibiotics. With the aid of such measures, infection rates in the UK between 1993 and 1996 fell to 1.08% [9].

5.3. Prophylaxis

Bacterial contamination of theatre air was initially recognized as a risk factor for post operative sepsis by Lister in 1867 [102]. Charnley later introduced the concept of ultraclean air flow ventilation that produces less than 10 colony forming units per cubic meter [103]. His reported infection rates in THA fell to 1% with the use of such enclosures. A MRC trial published in 1982 demonstrated a deep sepsis rate of 0.6% with ultraclean ventilation compared to 1.5% with conventional ventilation [104]. The use of ultraclean air ventilation during joint arthroplasty has subsequently become universally adopted practice within the UK [105].

The use of peri-operative antibiotics during THA is also a common prophylactic measure. Early trials using cloxacillin in THA found a 12% infection rate without prophylaxis compared to 0% with [106]. Currently cephalosporins are commonly used prophylaxis for THA. There is however a gradual move away from these due to the emergence of MRSA and problems with Clostridium difficile infection. Alternative regimens include flucloxacillin and gentamicin, or vancomycin and gentamicin. There is no conclusive evidence with regards to the optimal antibiotic regimen or duration of administration. However no benefit of extended prophylaxis beyond 24 hours has been demonstrated [107]. Therefore antibiotic regimes should be ideally guided by local microbiological knowledge so locally prevalent organisms can be targeted. Other measures shown to reduce rates of infection or bacterial load include the use of occlusive clothing, exhaust suits, pulsed wound lavage, preoperative showering and reducing theatre traffic [105].

5.4. Pathogenesis

Infection can arise by direct bacterial contamination at the time of surgery or later haematogenous spread. Staphylococcus aureus was the most common causative organism in an early series published by Charnley [108]. Coagulase negative staphylococci have become increasingly prevalent over the years with a recent series showing such organisms responsible for 58% of infections [109]. This is thought to be due to the effect of antibiotic use on bacterial flora [105]. Risk factors for periprosthetic infection include obesity, revision surgery, inflammatory arthritis, open skin lesions on the affected limb, blood transfusion, urinary infections and high ASA score [110].

Pathogenesis begins with bacterial adhesion. Primary adhesion occurs due to physical interactions (hydrophobic/electrostatic) between the bacteria and prosthetic surface. This is followed by bacterial aggregation through membrane adhesion molecules and generation of exopolysaccharides which form a glyocalyx or biofilm surrounding the bacteria [111]. This biofilm is thought to protect the bacteria from antibiotics and host defences [112].

5.5. Classification

Periprosthetic infections can be classified into 4 main catogeries [113]. Early postoperative infection is one that becomes apparent within one month of the procedure. Late chronic infection presents later than 1 month after operation and has an insidious course of gradual onset of pain and swelling with minimal systemic symptoms. Acute haematogenous spread results in an acute onset of symptoms associated with a documented or suspected bacteraemia. The final type is positive intra-operative culture, this is an occult infection diagnosed by positive cultures taken at time of revision surgery.

5.6. Diagnosis

Diagnosis of peri-prosthetic infection can be extremely challenging. Hip pain is the most consistent symptom. Presence of systemic symptoms such as fevers or rigors can be very variable. Examination may reveal local wound tenderness, signs of inflammation, discharge, sinuses and a painful range of movement.

Plain radiographs may show evidence of osteopenia or osteolysis, periostiitis and endosteal scalloping. However none of these can reliably differentiate between infection and aseptic loosening. Radionucleotide scanning using technetium or gallium can also been used. Technetium uptake reflects active bone turnover and gallium binds to transferrin, accumulating in inflammatory foci. Technetium scanning has a greater sensitivity than gallium for infection but their inability to differentiate infection and aseptic loosening limits their application [114, 115]. However its relatively high negative predictive value can make technetium bone scanning a useful initial screening test [116]. 18F-Fluoro-deoxyglucose [18-FDG] PET scanning is a newer technique that has increased sensitivity and specificity for infection. Pooled data from recent studies demonstrate a sensitivity of 85.5% and a specificity of 92.6% for periprosthetic infection [117]. Availability of PET scanners however still remains poor. Using radio-labelled white cells or immunoglobulins is another technique which has shown improved sensitivity and specificity relative to traditional three phase bone scans. Their widespread availability combined with the lack of established diagnostic criteria for 18-FDG PET scans, makes labelled white cell scans the current nuclear medicine investigation of choice for periprosthetic infection [118].

Blood investigations include ESR, CRP and Interleukin-6. ESR and CRP are non specific inflammatory markers and therefore can be elevated by concurrent illnesses. In the absence of such conditions an ESR greater than 30 mm/hr has a sensitivity and specificity of 82 and 85% respectively for peri-prosthetic infection, and the values for a CRP greater than 10mg/l are 96% and 92% [119]. Elevated levels of interleukin-6 have also been associated with periprosthetic infection with a sensitivity and specificity of 100% and 95% in one study [120]. However other chronic inflammatory conditions such as rheumatoid arthritis and other illnesses such as AIDS and Multiple Sclerosis can also cause elevated levels.

Cytological and microbiological analysis of hip aspirate taken under sterile conditions can give useful information regarding not only the presence of infection but also the potential offending organism. Ali et al. have shown a sensitivity and specificity of 0.82 and 0.91 for radiologically guided guided hip aspiration. However recent antibiotics can affect cultures and therefore antibiotics must be stopped for at least 2 weeks prior to aspiration.

5.7. Treatment

The aims of treatment of an infected prosthesis are eradication of infection and restoration of function. The classification by Tsukyama et al. can be used to help guide treatment [113]. Acute infections either presenting as early infection or acute haematogenous spread can be treated by component retention and thorough debridement, irrigation and intravenous antibiotics. However such treatment must be undertaken within 2 weeks of onset of symptoms [121]. Success rates between 50-74% have been reported with such a strategy [113].

Late chronic infection is best treated with full revision. This can be performed as a single stage exchange arthroplasty or a 2 stage exchange procedure. Originally described by Bucholz, a single stage procedure involves prosthesis removal, soft tissue debridement and lavage, followed by re-implantation of a new prosthesis if a clean uninfected bed is achieved, followed by appropriate antibiotic therapy [122]. Review of 1299 cases treated with single stage revision showed an 83% success rate at an average follow up of 4.8 years [123]. Factors associated with successful outcome were good general health of the patient, absence of wound complications after the primary procedure, methicillin sensitive organisms and infection with organisms sensitive to antibiotics within the cement [123]. Advantages of a single stage procedure include lower patient morbidity and lower incidence of complications such as fracture and dislocation. However 2 stage procedures have consistently demonstrated higher success rates compared to single stage procedures [124-128]. Thus 2 stage exchange still remains the most common strategy.

2 stage procedures involve initial prosthesis removal, soft tissue debridement and insertion of an antibiotic loaded cement spacer. This can be in the form of an articulating spacer allowing some range of movement and reducing soft tissue contracture. This is followed by

appropriate antibiotic therapy and a usual interval of 6 weeks prior to reimplantation of the definite new prosthesis. Success rates of between 87 to 94% have been reported with cemented 2 stage revision [124, 125, 128].

6. Nerve and vessel injury

The overall incidence of nerve injury after THA is estimated to be around 1% [129]. Sciatic nerve palsies account for 79% of all cases, followed by femoral nerve palsies (13%), combined femoral and sciatic nerve palsy (5.8%) and obturator nerve palsy (1.6%) [129]. In the majority of cases (47%) the aetiology is unknown. Other causes include traction (20%), contusion (19%), haematoma (11%) and dislocation (2%), with laceration only accounting for 1% of all nerve palsies [130]. Risk factors for nerve injury include female sex, revision surgery and developmental dysplasia of the acetabulum [129].

When the sciatic nerve is affected, it most commonly involves the common peroneal division. This is thought to be due to the lower amount of connective tissue present between the funiculi and its relatively tethered position at the sciatic notch compared to the tibial branch [129, 131]. These factors are thought to make the peroneal branch more susceptible to trauma and traction. The use of the posterior approach has traditionally been associated with increased risk of sciatic nerve damage. However a Cochrane review in 2006 found no difference in the incidence of nerve palsy between the posterior and direct lateral approaches [132]. Femoral nerve palsy is less common and is usually secondary to direct compression, usually due to a malpositioned retractor [130].

Indications for surgical intervention in a patient with nerve palsy include haematoma causing compression, palsy associated with excessive lengthening and palsy that can be definitely attributed to implanted metalwork. Electrodiagnostic studies can be helpful in determining the level of the lesion. Outcomes of nerve palsies are variable, with 40% of patients showing a good recovery, 45% of patients having mild residual motor or sensory symptoms and 15% left with a dense motor or sensory deficit [129]. Partial nerve lesions and maintenance of some motor function are good prognostic indicators, with recovery possible for up to 3 years after the initial insult [133].

Vascular injury during THA is extremely rare. Published incidence varies between 0.04 to 0.08% [134, 135]. As opposed to knee arthroplasty, vascular injury in THA is usually the result of direct trauma either during component insertion or removal [136]. Risk factors include revision surgery, previous vascular injury or surgery and pre-existing atherosclerosis [137]. The majority of vascular injuries are arterial but venous injury has been described [138]. Venous injuries however may be under diagnosed as they may run a relatively benign course remaining undetected.

The majority of vascular injuries are either the result direct trauma from acetabular retractors or acetabular screw insertion [130]. Wasielewski et al. have described an acetabular quadrant system to help guide safe screw insertion [139]. The postero-superior and poster-inferior quadrants are the safest zones for screw insertion as they have they areas of greatest bone stock [139].

6.1. Wear and aseptic loosening

Aseptic loosening is the most common cause for revision surgery, accounting for 75% of revision cases [140]. Aseptic failure occurs as a result of a chronic inflammatory reaction secondary to particulate wear debris eventually resulting in osteoclast activation, osteolysis and loosening [141].

The pathogenesis begins with the generation of wear particles from the bearing surface, and also non bearing surfaces such as the interface between acetabular shell and the liner insert, known as backside wear. The morphology of the wear debris is dependent on the type of implant used. Particles from polyethylene bearing surfaces can vary from submicron in size to several millimetres. The average size of polyethylene debris has been shown to be around 0.5 μm and it is this submicron sized particle that has been shown to have the most bio-reactivity [142, 143]. The rate of generation of the wear particles has also been shown to correlate with the degree of osteolysis [142]. Inadequate initial fixation can also contribute to loosening by generating micromotion and increasing the rate of generation of particulate debris [144]. This highlights the importance of good cementation techniques in reducing the risk of aseptic failure. Pressure within the joint fluid has also been suggested to contribute to osteolysis. Increased joint fluid pressure in animal models has been shown to induce bone loss at the prosthesis bone interface possibly by interfering with bone perfusion causing osteocyte death [145, 146]. Increased joint fluid pressures have been noted in THAs undergoing revision and pressure waves generated by load bearing have been demonstrated in retroacetabular lytic lesions [147, 148]. Thus increased fluid pressures may directly contribute to osteolysis and also perpetuate the dissemination of the wear debris throughout the prosthesis bone interface, enhancing the biological response.

The primary response to wear debris is predominantly macrophage mediated. The exact mechanism of macrophage activation is still unclear. Macrophages can be activated as a result of either phagocytosis of particulate matter and also possibly through cell membrane interactions with particulate matter [149]. Macrophage activation causes the release of proinflammatory cytokines and growth factors including TNF-α, Interleukin-1, TGF-β and RANKL [150]. This results in the production of a pseudomembrane at the bone cement prosthesis interface consisting of macrophages, fibroblasts and lymphocytes within a connective tissue matrix [151]. TNF-α and Interleukin-1 both promote osteoclastic differentiation and activation, but it is the up regulation of the RANK/RANKL pathway that is the key to activating osteoclastogenesis and subsequent osteolysis [143]. Recent studies have suggested individual genetic susceptibility to osteolysis may exist via single nucleotide polymorphisms in the implicated cytokine genes, possibly by altering the magnitude of the biological response [152-155].

Alternative bearing surfaces can be used to reduce wear rates, debris generation and subsequent osteolysis. Highly crosslinked polyethylene, ceramic on ceramic and metal on metal bearings have all been shown to have reduced wear rates compared to standard ultra-high molecular weight polyethylene (UHWPE) [156-164]. However there are concerns regarding the increased bioreactivity of crosslinked polyethylene debris compared to standard UHWPE which may offset the benefits of reduced volumetric wear [165, 166]. Volumetric wear is also lower with metal on metal bearings. However as the particle size is much smaller, usually between 20-90nm, the overall surface area is much larger compared to UHWPE raising concerns of possible increased bioreactivity.

Pain is usually the primary presenting symptom of aseptic failure. Gross acetabular loosening can cause groin pain whereas thigh pain can indicate femoral loosening [167]. Early loosening however may also be asymptomatic merely detected on routine follow up radiographs. Clinical signs may include inability to straight leg raise, shortening of the leg due to subsidence and increasing external rotation of the leg if the femoral stem twists into retroversion. Investigations for aseptic loosening are similar to those for infection discussed earlier. Blood inflammatory markers such as CRP are usually normal with aseptic loosening [168]. Radiological tests include plain radiography, subtraction and nuclear arthrography and bone scintigraphy. Meta-analysis has shown similar diagnostic performance for all of these tests and therefore suggests plain radiographs and bone scintigraphy as the tests of choice due to their lower risk of patient morbidity [169]. CT 3D imaging is also useful for the evaluation of lytic lesions as plain 2 dimensional radiographs can underestimate the size of the lesion as demonstrated in figure 1 [170, 171].

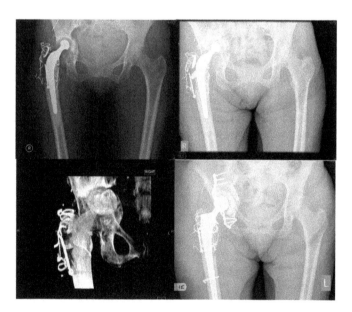

Figure 6. Top left & right, Progressive acetabular osteolysis over 1.5 years, **Bottom left,** 3D CT reconstruction demonstrating lesion and pelvic discontinuity, **Bottom right,** defect reconstructed with mesh and bone graft and plate to posterior column to address discontinuity

Treatment of aseptic loosening is guided by the severity of the patient's symptoms and the rate and volume of osteolysis. Indications for surgical treatment in asymptomatic patients are progressive osteolysis and risk of catastrophic mechanical failure such as periprosthetic fracture. Nonsurgical treatment using bisphosphonates and anti cytokine therapy such as anti-TNF-α to prevent progression of osteolysis has been suggested. However their efficacy is yet to be determined [172]. Goals of surgical treatment include removal of wear debris and also the wear generator, reconstruction of the osseous lesion and restoration of mechanical stability [173]. This can involve exchange of bearing surfaces, bone grafting of lytic lesions and revision of loose components.

7. Bearing specific complications

7.1. Ceramic on ceramic bearings

Ceramic articulations have become increasingly popular due to their low wear profile and good biocompatibility. However potential complications of ceramic bearings include chipping and incomplete seating of ceramic liners during insertion, fracture and bearing generated noise.

Currently all ceramic acetabular bearings consist of a modular ceramic liner which is inserted into a metal shell implanted into the acetabulum. Incomplete seating of the liner due to soft tissue interposition or deformation of the metal shell has been reported [174, 175]. Thus extra care and good visualisation of the acetabulum is imperative when inserting a modular ceramic liner. Chipping during impaction has also been reported and this can also be secondary to deformation of the metal shell [176]. Using titanium sleeved or recessed ceramic liners has been shown to reduce such risks [177].

Risk of fracture for modern 3rd generation ceramic bearings is extremely low. Willman et al. found a fracture rate of 0.004% for femoral heads manufactured after 1994 [178]. Fracture of both the liner and femoral head have however been reported [179, 180]. Head fracture has been associated with improper handling during implantation. Contamination of the stemball interface with blood or soft tissue has been shown to significantly reduce the load required for inducing fracture [181]. Impingement of the femoral neck on the edge of ceramics liner is thought to be a major risk factor for liner fracture [179, 182]. Therefore correct positioning of the acetabular component is especially important for ceramic bearings.

Noise generated from ceramic bearings is a recently described phenomenon. Published rates of "squeaky" ceramic bearings range from 2.7% to 20.9% [183, 184]. Component malposition has been implicated [185]. However recent studies have found no association between cup inclination and version and the incidence of squeaking [183, 184]. Short neck length is the only factor that has been associated with squeaking, possibly due to impingement or microseperation to due increased joint laxity [184]. Revision of squeaking hips has revealed evidence of stripe wear but there is currently no evidence to suggest squeaking is a precursor for ceramic fracture [186, 187].

7.2. Metal on metal bearings

Metal on metal bearings also have superior wear rates compared to standard UHMWPE [161, 163, 164]. However there is increasing concern regarding metal ion toxicity and hypersensitivity type reactions. Volumetric wear is considerably lower for metal bearings compared to UHMWPE, but the absolute number of particles generated is estimated to be 13500 times higher [188]. Therefore the total surface area is considerably higher. Thus the bioreactivity of metal wear particles may be higher than polyethylene or ceramic debris, and the nanometre scale of the particles and dissolution of metal ions allows distant transport, raising concerns of systemic toxicity.

The possibility of systemic toxicity has raised interest in serum metal ion levels in patients with modern metal on metal bearings. Recent studies using standardised measurement techniques have reported mean serum chromium levels of between 0.86 – 17.7 µg/L [189-192]. Safe levels of serum metal ion levels have however yet to be determined [193]. Concerns regarding carcinogenesis and immune suppression secondary to raised blood metal ion levels have been raised [194, 195]. Teratogenicity is also another potential concern as transplacental crossage of metal ions has been demonstrated [196]. However, currently no conclusive evidence exists supporting these theories [197, 198]. A positive correlation between cup inclination and blood metal ion levels has been demonstrated with metal on metal bearings [191, 199]. This is probably due to increased edge loading with increasing cup inclination and serum metal ion levels have been suggested as a tool to monitor the performance of metal on metal bearings [190]. Therefore metal ion exposure can be minimised with proper cup orientation.

Local tissue reactions to metal on metal articulations have also been reported [200-202]. Metal ions are thought to induce an immune reaction leading to tissue necrosis and osteolysis. This is in contrast to UHMWPE which induces a macrophage reaction to particulate wear debris. Willert et al. has called this unique reaction, aseptic lymphocytic vasculitic associated lesions (ALVAL) [200]. Histologically this reaction is characterised by perivascular lymphocytic infiltration and plasma cells. Clinical presentation can vary between chronic groin pain to extensive tissue necrosis forming pseudotumours [201]. Exact incidence of such tissue reactions is unknown but is estimated to be around 1% [201]. Risk factors associated with the development of these adverse reactions include small component size and component malposition [203]. Stemmed metal on metal hip replacements also appear to have a higher rate of revision and their use has now been discouraged [204].

8. Periprosthetic fracture

Periprosthetic fractures can occur either intraoperatively or in the postoperative period. Overall, periprosthetic fractures more commonly affect the femoral component of the THA. Data from the largest published series by Berry et al. reports the incidence of intra- and postoperative femoral fracture as 1% and 1.1% respectively [13]. Rates of intraoperative fracture after cementless fixation are higher, 5.4% for primary THAs and 21% for revision surgery [13].

The treatment of unstable postoperative periprosthetic femoral fractures is now almost always operative. Loosening, non-union, varus malunion and morbidity associated with prolonged immobility have made conservative management unpopular [205]. Treatment can be guided by using the Vancouver classification which is the most widely accepted system for classifying such fractures [206]. This system takes into account three main factors, site of the fracture, stability of the implant and quality of the surrounding bone. Type A fractures occur in the trochanteric region and are subdivided into type A_G and A_L fractures. A_G fractures involve the greater trochanter and usually stable and can therefore be treated conservatively with protected weightbearing. A_L fractures involve the lesser trochanter, and are also usually insignificant unless a large portion of the calcar is involved potentially affecting implant stability, in which case revision THA may be necessary. Type B fractures occur around or just distal to the stem and are subdivided into type B_1, B_2 and B_3 fractures. B_1 fractures have a well fixed stem and can be treated with open reduction and internal fixation. Combined plate and cerclage wire systems are commonly used for such fractures. Type B_2 fractures have a loose stem but good bone stock. These are usually revised with long stem implants bypassing the fracture, and can be augmented by plates, cables and strut allografts to improve stability. Type B_3 fractures have a loose stem and poor stock stock. These are the most difficult to treat and require either revision THA with structural allografts to reconstitute the proximal femur, distally fixed long stemmed implants of custom proximal femoral replacement. Type C fractures occur distal to the stem. The stem can therefore essentially be ignored and the fracture treated with standard open reduction and internal fixation.

Acetabular fractures are somewhat less common with reported intraoperative rates ranging between 0.02-0.4% [207, 208]. Data regarding postoperative fractures is currently not available [13]. The majority of intraoperative acetabular fractures occur during acetabular insertion especially during impaction of pressfit cementless components [209]. Underreaming by greater than 2mm has been suggested to significantly increase fracture risk [210].

The aims of treatment of intraoperative acetabular fractures include stabilizing the fracture and preventing further propagation and maintaining component stability [209]. Techniques include plating the anterior and posterior columns and using bone graft and jumbo revision cups if there is marked bone loss. Treatment of postoperative fractures follows similar principles. Early postoperative fractures with stable cups and minimally displaced fractures, especially around uncemented implants with supplemental screw fixation, can be treated conservatively. Unstable cups require revision with fixation of the fracture. Late presenting fractures are frequently associated with osteolysis and therefore usually require revision with bone grafting [211].

9. Heterotopic ossification

Heterotopic ossification (HO) is the abnormal formation of mature lamellar bone within extraskeletal soft tissues. HO is most commonly asymptomatic, merely detected on follow up radiology. When symptomatic, stiffness is the most common presentation. Pain and soft tissue signs such as localised warmth, mild oedema and erythema are uncommon but can cause confusion raising concerns over infection [212].

Early changes of HO within the soft tissues can be detected after 3 weeks on bone scan and plain radiographic changes can take 6 weeks to become apparent [212]. Extensive bone deposition can occur within 3 months, but full maturation takes up to one year [213]. The abductor compartment is most commonly affected. HO is most commonly classified using the Brooker classification [214]. This is based upon plain anteroposterior radiographs of the pelvis and is outlined in figure 7.

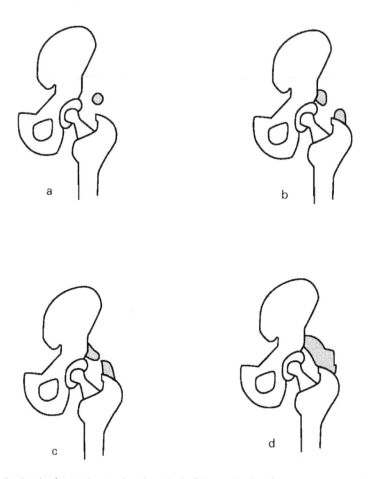

Figure 7. Brooker classification showing a) grade 1: islands of bone within the soft tissues about the hip, b) grade 2: bony spurs from either the femur or the pelvis, with a gap of more than 1 cm between opposing bony ends, c) grade 3: the gaps between the spurs are less than 1 cm and d) grade 4: apparent ankylosis of the hip due to the heterotopic ossification.

The pathophysiology is believed to involve inappropriate differentiation of pluripotent mesenchymal stem cells into osteoblasts, causing the excess bone formation [215]. Overexpression of bone morphogenetic protein-4 has been implicated [216, 217].

Incidence of clinically significant HO is reported to be between 3 – 7% [218, 219]. Risk factors include male gender, previous history of HO, pre-existing hip fusion, hypertrophic osteoarthritis, ankylosing spondylitis, diffuse idiopathic skeletal hyperostosis, Paget's disease, post traumatic osteoarthritis, osteonecrosis and rheumatoid arthritis [14]. Surgical factors include extensive soft tissue dissection, haematoma and persistence of bone debris. Evidence implicating the role of surgical approach is debatable [14].

Treatment of symptomatic patients can initially involve intensive physiotherapy during the maturation phase. The efficacy of this treatment is however yet to be determined. Surgical management involves excision of the HO after maturation of the bone is allowed, followed by appropriate prophylaxis. Improvements in range of motion in all planes has been reported with surgical excision [220].

Patients at high risk of HO should be given prophylaxis either in the form of non steroidal anti-inflammatory medication (NSAIDs) or radiotherapy. Preoperative radiotherapy, 4 hours before, or post operative radiotherapy within 72 hours has been shown to be the most effective method of prophylaxis [221-223]. This involves a single dose of between 7 – 8 Gy. Combination therapy with NSAIDs and radiotherapy can be considered in patients at highest risk of HO such as patients undergoing excision of symptomatic HO [14].

10. Conclusion

- Complications following total hip arthroplasty can be classified into procedure specific or systemic. On the whole complication rates have fallen with time due to improved surgical and anaesthetic technique.

- The most common symptomatic systemic complication is DVT and data suggests that DVT rates post THA have not fallen with time.

- The most common cause for revision is aseptic loosening. Registry data suggests up to 75% of revision surgery may be due to aseptic loosening.

- Infection is one of the most feared complications. Rates with prophylactic measures such as antibiotics and clean air enclosures have however dropped significantly to below 1%.

- Leg length discrepancy is one of the most common causes of patient dissatisfaction and is the most common cause of litigation in the USA.

Despite the potential wide range of complication that can occur after THA, it remains one of the most successful orthopaedic interventions

List of abbreviations used

THA: Total Hip Arthroplasty

DVT: Deep Vein Thrombosis

PE: Pulmonary Embolism

THA: Total Hip Arthroplasty

PLAD: Posterior Lip Augmentation Device

UHMWPE: Ultra High Molecular Weight Polyehtylene

LLD: Limb Length Discrepancy

TGF-β: Transforming Growth Factor – Beta

RANKL: Receptor activator of nuclear factor kappa-B ligand

UHMWPE: Ultra High Molecular Weight Polyethylene

TNF-α: Tumour Necrosis Factor – Alpha

ALVAL: aseptic lymphocytic vasculitic associated lesions

HO: Heterotopic Ossification

Author details

Asim Rajpura and Tim Board*

*Address all correspondence to: tim@timboard.co.uk

Wrightington Hospital, Hall Lane, Appley Bridge, Wigan, Lancashire, UK

References

[1] Registry NJ. Summary of annual statistics (England and Wales). National Joint Registry 2009 [cited 2009 04/02/2009].

[2] Jones CA, Voaklander DC, Johnston DW, Suarez-Almazor ME. Health related quality of life outcomes after total hip and knee arthroplasties in a community based population. J Rheumatol. 2000 Jul;27(7):1745-52.

[3] Mancuso CA, Salvati EA, Johanson NA, Peterson MG, Charlson ME. Patients' expectations and satisfaction with total hip arthroplasty. J Arthroplasty. 1997 Jun;12(4): 387-96.

[4] Liu SS, Gonzalez Della Valle A, Besculides MC, Gaber LK, Memtsoudis SG. Trends in mortality, complications, and demographics for primary hip arthroplasty in the United States. Int Orthop. 2008 May 7.

[5] Pitto RP, Koessler M. The risk of fat embolism during cemented total hip replacement in the elderly patient. Chir Organi Mov. 1999 Apr-Jun;84(2):119-28.

[6] Kwon MS, Kuskowski M, Mulhall KJ, Macaulay W, Brown TE, Saleh KJ. Does surgical approach affect total hip arthroplasty dislocation rates? Clin Orthop Relat Res. 2006 Jun;447:34-8.

[7] Wylde V, Whitehouse SL, Taylor AH, Pattison GT, Bannister GC, Blom AW. Prevalence and functional impact of patient-perceived leg length discrepancy after hip replacement. Int Orthop. 2008 Apr 25.

[8] Samama CM, Ravaud P, Parent F, Barre J, Mertl P, Mismetti P. Epidemiology of venous thromboembolism after lower limb arthroplasty: the FOTO study. J Thromb Haemost. 2007 Dec;5(12):2360-7.

[9] Blom AW, Taylor AH, Pattison G, Whitehouse S, Bannister GC. Infection after total hip arthroplasty. The Avon experience. J Bone Joint Surg Br. 2003 Sep;85(7):956-9.

[10] Mantilla CB, Horlocker TT, Schroeder DR, Berry DJ, Brown DL. Frequency of myocardial infarction, pulmonary embolism, deep venous thrombosis, and death following primary hip or knee arthroplasty. Anesthesiology. 2002 May;96(5):1140-6.

[11] Hallan G, Lie SA, Furnes O, Engesaeter LB, Vollset SE, Havelin LI. Medium- and long-term performance of 11,516 uncemented primary femoral stems from the Norwegian arthroplasty register. J Bone Joint Surg Br. 2007 Dec;89(12):1574-80.

[12] Ling RS, Charity J, Lee AJ, Whitehouse SL, Timperley AJ, Gie GA. The long-term results of the original exeter polished cemented femoral component a follow-up report. J Arthroplasty. 2009 Jun;24(4):511-7.

[13] Berry DJ. Epidemiology: hip and knee. Orthop Clin North Am. 1999 Apr;30(2): 183-90.

[14] Board TN, Karva A, Board RE, Gambhir AK, Porter ML. The prophylaxis and treatment of heterotopic ossification following lower limb arthroplasty. J Bone Joint Surg Br. 2007 Apr;89(4):434-40.

[15] Kim YH, Oh SH, Kim JS. Incidence and natural history of deep-vein thrombosis after total hip arthroplasty. A prospective and randomised clinical study. J Bone Joint Surg Br. 2003 Jul;85(5):661-5.

[16] NICE. Venous thromboembolism: reducing the risk of venous thromboembolism (deep vein thrombosis and pulmonary embolism) in inpatients undergoing surgery: National Collaborating Centre for Acute Care; 2007.

[17] Xing KH, Morrison G, Lim W, Douketis J, Odueyungbo A, Crowther M. Has the incidence of deep vein thrombosis in patients undergoing total hip/knee arthroplasty

changed over time? A systematic review of randomized controlled trials. Thromb Res. 2008;123(1):24-34.

[18] Sharrock NE, Go G, Harpel PC, Ranawat CS, Sculco TP, Salvati EA. The John Charnley Award. Thrombogenesis during total hip arthroplasty. Clin Orthop Relat Res. 1995 Oct(319):16-27.

[19] Borghi B, Casati A. Thromboembolic complications after total hip replacement. Int Orthop. 2002;26(1):44-7.

[20] McNally MA, Mollan RA. Total hip replacement, lower limb blood flow and venous thrombogenesis. J Bone Joint Surg Br. 1993 Jul;75(4):640-4.

[21] Beksac B, Gonzalez Della Valle A, Salvati EA. Thromboembolic disease after total hip arthroplasty: who is at risk? Clin Orthop Relat Res. 2006 Dec;453:211-24.

[22] Modig J, Hjelmstedt A, Sahlstedt B, Maripuu E. Comparative influences of epidural and general anaesthesia on deep venous thrombosis and pulmonary embolism after total hip replacement. Acta Chir Scand. 1981;147(2):125-30.

[23] Davis FM, Laurenson VG, Gillespie WJ, Wells JE, Foate J, Newman E. Deep vein thrombosis after total hip replacement. A comparison between spinal and general anaesthesia. J Bone Joint Surg Br. 1989 Mar;71(2):181-5.

[24] Davis FM, Laurenson VG, Gillespie WJ, Foate J, Seagar AD. Leg blood flow during total hip replacement under spinal or general anaesthesia. Anaesth Intensive Care. 1989 May;17(2):136-43.

[25] Stannard JP, Harris RM, Bucknell AL, Cossi A, Ward J, Arrington ED. Prophylaxis of deep venous thrombosis after total hip arthroplasty by using intermittent compression of the plantar venous plexus. Am J Orthop. 1996 Feb;25(2):127-34.

[26] Ryan MG, Westrich GH, Potter HG, Sharrock N, Maun LM, Macaulay W, et al. Effect of mechanical compression on the prevalence of proximal deep venous thrombosis as assessed by magnetic resonance venography. J Bone Joint Surg Am. 2002 Nov;84-A(11):1998-2004.

[27] Zufferey P, Laporte S, Quenet S, Molliex S, Auboyer C, Decousus H, et al. Optimal low-molecular-weight heparin regimen in major orthopaedic surgery. A meta-analysis of randomised trials. Thromb Haemost. 2003 Oct;90(4):654-61.

[28] Lassen MR, Borris LC, Anderson BS, Jensen HP, Skejo Bro HP, Andersen G, et al. Efficacy and safety of prolonged thromboprophylaxis with a low molecular weight heparin (dalteparin) after total hip arthroplasty--the Danish Prolonged Prophylaxis (DaPP) Study. Thromb Res. 1998 Mar 15;89(6):281-7.

[29] Turpie AG, Bauer KA, Eriksson BI, Lassen MR. Fondaparinux vs enoxaparin for the prevention of venous thromboembolism in major orthopedic surgery: a meta-analysis of 4 randomized double-blind studies. Arch Intern Med. 2002 Sep 9;162(16):1833-40.

[30] Lassen MR, Bauer KA, Eriksson BI, Turpie AG. Postoperative fondaparinux versus preoperative enoxaparin for prevention of venous thromboembolism in elective hip-replacement surgery: a randomised double-blind comparison. Lancet. 2002 May 18;359(9319):1715-20.

[31] Pitto RP, Hamer H, Heiss-Dunlop W, Kuehle J. Mechanical prophylaxis of deep-vein thrombosis after total hip replacement a randomised clinical trial. J Bone Joint Surg Br. 2004 Jul;86(5):639-42.

[32] Kakkar VV, Howes J, Sharma V, Kadziola Z. A comparative double-blind, randomised trial of a new second generation LMWH (bemiparin) and UFH in the prevention of post-operative venous thromboembolism. The Bemiparin Assessment group. Thromb Haemost. 2000 Apr;83(4):523-9.

[33] Dahl OE, Andreassen G, Aspelin T, Muller C, Mathiesen P, Nyhus S, et al. Prolonged thromboprophylaxis following hip replacement surgery--results of a double-blind, prospective, randomised, placebo-controlled study with dalteparin (Fragmin). Thromb Haemost. 1997 Jan;77(1):26-31.

[34] Turpie AG, Eriksson BI, Lassen MR, Bauer KA. A meta-analysis of fondaparinux versus enoxaparin in the prevention of venous thromboembolism after major orthopaedic surgery. J South Orthop Assoc. 2002 Winter;11(4):182-8.

[35] Eriksson BI, Borris LC, Friedman RJ, Haas S, Huisman MV, Kakkar AK, et al. Rivaroxaban versus enoxaparin for thromboprophylaxis after hip arthroplasty. N Engl J Med. 2008 Jun 26;358(26):2765-75.

[36] Kakkar AK, Brenner B, Dahl OE, Eriksson BI, Mouret P, Muntz J, et al. Extended duration rivaroxaban versus short-term enoxaparin for the prevention of venous thromboembolism after total hip arthroplasty: a double-blind, randomised controlled trial. Lancet. 2008 Jul 5;372(9632):31-9.

[37] Raskob GE, Gallus AS, Pineo GF, Chen D, Ramirez LM, Wright RT, et al. Apixaban versus enoxaparin for thromboprophylaxis after hip or knee replacement: pooled analysis of major venous thromboembolism and bleeding in 8464 patients from the ADVANCE-2 and ADVANCE-3 trials. J Bone Joint Surg Br. 2012 Feb;94(2):257-64.

[38] Jensen CD, Steval A, Partington PF, Reed MR, Muller SD. Return to theatre following total hip and knee replacement, before and after the introduction of rivaroxaban: a retrospective cohort study. J Bone Joint Surg Br. 2011 Jan;93(1):91-5.

[39] NICE. Venous thromboembolism, reducing the risk of venous thromboembolism (deep vein thrombosis and pulmonary embolism) in patients admitted to hospital. London: National Clinical Guideline Centre; 2010.

[40] Pulido L, Parvizi J, Macgibeny M, Sharkey PF, Purtill JJ, Rothman RH, et al. In hospital complications after total joint arthroplasty. J Arthroplasty. 2008 Sep;23(6 Suppl 1): 139-45.

[41] Roderick P, Ferris G, Wilson K, Halls H, Jackson D, Collins R, et al. Towards evidence-based guidelines for the prevention of venous thromboembolism: systematic reviews of mechanical methods, oral anticoagulation, dextran and regional anaesthesia as thromboprophylaxis. Health Technol Assess. 2005 Dec;9(49):iii-iv, ix-x, 1-78.

[42] Haas S, Breyer HG, Bacher HP, Fareed J, Misselwitz F, Victor N, et al. Prevention of major venous thromboembolism following total hip or knee replacement: a randomized comparison of low-molecular-weight heparin with unfractionated heparin (ECHOS Trial). Int Angiol. 2006 Dec;25(4):335-42.

[43] Hooker JA, Lachiewicz PF, Kelley SS. Efficacy of prophylaxis against thromboembolism with intermittent pneumatic compression after primary and revision total hip arthroplasty. J Bone Joint Surg Am. 1999 May;81(5):690-6.

[44] Eriksson BI, Kalebo P, Anthymyr BA, Wadenvik H, Tengborn L, Risberg B. Prevention of deep-vein thrombosis and pulmonary embolism after total hip replacement. Comparison of low-molecular-weight heparin and unfractionated heparin. J Bone Joint Surg Am. 1991 Apr;73(4):484-93.

[45] Handoll HH, Farrar MJ, McBirnie J, Tytherleigh-Strong G, Milne AA, Gillespie WJ. Heparin, low molecular weight heparin and physical methods for preventing deep vein thrombosis and pulmonary embolism following surgery for hip fractures. Cochrane Database Syst Rev. 2002(4):CD000305.

[46] Fender D, Harper WM, Thompson JR, Gregg PJ. Mortality and fatal pulmonary embolism after primary total hip replacement. Results from a regional hip register. J Bone Joint Surg Br. 1997 Nov;79(6):896-9.

[47] Joels CS, Sing RF, Heniford BT. Complications of inferior vena cava filters. Am Surg. 2003 Aug;69(8):654-9.

[48] Kallos T, Enis JE, Gollan F, Davis JH. Intramedullary pressure and pulmonary embolism of femoral medullary contents in dogs during insertion of bone cement and a prosthesis. J Bone Joint Surg Am. 1974 Oct;56(7):1363-7.

[49] Tronzo RG, Kallos T, Wyche MQ. Elevation of intramedullary pressure when methylmethacrylate is inserted in total hip arthroplasty. J Bone Joint Surg Am. 1974 Jun; 56(4):714-8.

[50] Wenda K, Degreif J, Runkel M, Ritter G. Pathogenesis and prophylaxis of circulatory reactions during total hip replacement. Arch Orthop Trauma Surg. 1993;112(6):260-5.

[51] Colonna DM, Kilgus D, Brown W, Challa V, Stump DA, Moody DM. Acute brain fat embolization occurring after total hip arthroplasty in the absence of a patent foramen ovale. Anesthesiology. 2002 Apr;96(4):1027-9.

[52] Forteza AM, Koch S, Romano JG, Zych G, Bustillo IC, Duncan RC, et al. Transcranial doppler detection of fat emboli. Stroke. 1999 Dec;30(12):2687-91.

[53] Edmonds CR, Barbut D, Hager D, Sharrock NE. Intraoperative cerebral arterial embolization during total hip arthroplasty. Anesthesiology. 2000 Aug;93(2):315-8.

[54] Memtsoudis SG, Rosenberger P, Walz JM. Critical care issues in the patient after major joint replacement. J Intensive Care Med. 2007 Mar-Apr;22(2):92-104.

[55] Christie J, Robinson CM, Singer B, Ray DC. Medullary lavage reduces embolic phenomena and cardiopulmonary changes during cemented hemiarthroplasty. J Bone Joint Surg Br. 1995 May;77(3):456-9.

[56] Pitto RP, Kossler M, Draenert K. [Prevention of fat and bone marrow embolism in cemented total hip endoprosthesis with vacuum cement technique]. Z Orthop Ihre Grenzgeb. 1998 Jul-Aug;136(4):Oa24.

[57] Aynardi M, Pulido L, Parvizi J, Sharkey PF, Rothman RH. Early mortality after modern total hip arthroplasty. Clin Orthop Relat Res. 2009 Jan;467(1):213-8.

[58] Kreder HJ, Berry GK, McMurtry IA, Halman SI. Arthroplasty in the octogenarian: quantifying the risks. J Arthroplasty. 2005 Apr;20(3):289-93.

[59] Eagle KA, Berger PB, Calkins H, Chaitman BR, Ewy GA, Fleischmann KE, et al. ACC/AHA Guideline Update for Perioperative Cardiovascular Evaluation for Noncardiac Surgery--Executive Summary. A report of the American College of Cardiology/American Heart Association Task Force on Practice Guidelines (Committee to Update the 1996 Guidelines on Perioperative Cardiovascular Evaluation for Noncardiac Surgery). Anesth Analg. 2002 May;94(5):1052-64.

[60] Moller AM, Pedersen T, Villebro N, Munksgaard A. Effect of smoking on early complications after elective orthopaedic surgery. J Bone Joint Surg Br. 2003 Mar;85(2): 178-81.

[61] Greenfield S, Apolone G, McNeil BJ, Cleary PD. The importance of co-existent disease in the occurrence of postoperative complications and one-year recovery in patients undergoing total hip replacement. Comorbidity and outcomes after hip replacement. Med Care. 1993 Feb;31(2):141-54.

[62] Parker MJ, Handoll HH, Griffiths R. Anaesthesia for hip fracture surgery in adults. Cochrane Database Syst Rev. 2001(4):CD000521.

[63] Sculco TP, Ranawat C. The use of spinal anesthesia for total hip-replacement arthroplasty. J Bone Joint Surg Am. 1975 Mar;57(2):173-7.

[64] O'Hara DA, Duff A, Berlin JA, Poses RM, Lawrence VA, Huber EC, et al. The effect of anesthetic technique on postoperative outcomes in hip fracture repair. Anesthesiology. 2000 Apr;92(4):947-57.

[65] Skutek M, Bourne RB, MacDonald SJ. (i) International epidemiology of revision THR. Current Orthopaedics. 2006;20(3):157-61.

[66] Patel PD, Potts A, Froimson MI. The dislocating hip arthroplasty: prevention and treatment. J Arthroplasty. 2007 Jun;22(4 Suppl 1):86-90.

[67] Sanchez-Sotelo J, Berry DJ. Epidemiology of instability after total hip replacement. Orthop Clin North Am. 2001 Oct;32(4):543-52, vii.

[68] Woo RY, Morrey BF. Dislocations after total hip arthroplasty. J Bone Joint Surg Am. 1982 Dec;64(9):1295-306.

[69] von Knoch M, Berry DJ, Harmsen WS, Morrey BF. Late dislocation after total hip arthroplasty. J Bone Joint Surg Am. 2002 Nov;84-A(11):1949-53.

[70] Soong M, Rubash HE, Macaulay W. Dislocation after total hip arthroplasty. J Am Acad Orthop Surg. 2004 Sep-Oct;12(5):314-21.

[71] Lee BP, Berry DJ, Harmsen WS, Sim FH. Total hip arthroplasty for the treatment of an acute fracture of the femoral neck: long-term results. J Bone Joint Surg Am. 1998 Jan;80(1):70-5.

[72] Goldstein WM, Gleason TF, Kopplin M, Branson JJ. Prevalence of dislocation after total hip arthroplasty through a posterolateral approach with partial capsulotomy and capsulorrhaphy. J Bone Joint Surg Am. 2001;83-A Suppl 2(Pt 1):2-7.

[73] White RE, Jr., Forness TJ, Allman JK, Junick DW. Effect of posterior capsular repair on early dislocation in primary total hip replacement. Clin Orthop Relat Res. 2001 Dec(393):163-7.

[74] Fackler CD, Poss R. Dislocation in total hip arthroplasties. Clin Orthop Relat Res. 1980 Sep(151):169-78.

[75] Lewinnek GE, Lewis JL, Tarr R, Compere CL, Zimmerman JR. Dislocations after total hip-replacement arthroplasties. J Bone Joint Surg Am. 1978 Mar;60(2):217-20.

[76] Barrack RL, Lavernia C, Ries M, Thornberry R, Tozakoglou E. Virtual reality computer animation of the effect of component position and design on stability after total hip arthroplasty. Orthop Clin North Am. 2001 Oct;32(4):569-77, vii.

[77] Nishii T, Sugano N, Miki H, Koyama T, Takao M, Yoshikawa H. Influence of component positions on dislocation: computed tomographic evaluations in a consecutive series of total hip arthroplasty. J Arthroplasty. 2004 Feb;19(2):162-6.

[78] Archbold HA, Mockford B, Molloy D, McConway J, Ogonda L, Beverland D. The transverse acetabular ligament: an aid to orientation of the acetabular component during primary total hip replacement: a preliminary study of 1000 cases investigating postoperative stability. J Bone Joint Surg Br. 2006 Jul;88(7):883-6.

[79] Amuwa C, Dorr LD. The combined anteversion technique for acetabular component anteversion. J Arthroplasty. 2008 Oct;23(7):1068-70.

[80] Barsoum WK, Patterson RW, Higuera C, Klika AK, Krebs VE, Molloy R. A computer model of the position of the combined component in the prevention of impingement in total hip replacement. J Bone Joint Surg Br. 2007 Jun;89(6):839-45.

[81] Kluess D, Martin H, Mittelmeier W, Schmitz KP, Bader R. Influence of femoral head size on impingement, dislocation and stress distribution in total hip replacement. Med Eng Phys. 2007 May;29(4):465-71.

[82] Burroughs BR, Hallstrom B, Golladay GJ, Hoeffel D, Harris WH. Range of motion and stability in total hip arthroplasty with 28-, 32-, 38-, and 44-mm femoral head sizes. J Arthroplasty. 2005 Jan;20(1):11-9.

[83] Bartz RL, Nobel PC, Kadakia NR, Tullos HS. The effect of femoral component head size on posterior dislocation of the artificial hip joint. J Bone Joint Surg Am. 2000 Sep; 82(9):1300-7.

[84] Bystrom S, Espehaug B, Furnes O, Havelin LI. Femoral head size is a risk factor for total hip luxation: a study of 42,987 primary hip arthroplasties from the Norwegian Arthroplasty Register. Acta Orthop Scand. 2003 Oct;74(5):514-24.

[85] Conroy JL, Whitehouse SL, Graves SE, Pratt NL, Ryan P, Crawford RW. Risk factors for revision for early dislocation in total hip arthroplasty. J Arthroplasty. 2008 Sep; 23(6):867-72.

[86] Hedlundh U, Ahnfelt L, Hybbinette CH, Wallinder L, Weckstrom J, Fredin H. Dislocations and the femoral head size in primary total hip arthroplasty. Clin Orthop Relat Res. 1996 Dec(333):226-33.

[87] Battaglia TC, Mulhall KJ, Brown TE, Saleh KJ. Increased surgical volume is associated with lower THA dislocation rates. Clin Orthop Relat Res. 2006 Jun;447:28-33.

[88] Schuh A, Mittelmeier W, Zeiler G, Behrend D, Kircher J, Bader R. Severe damage of the femoral head after dislocation and difficult reduction maneuvers after total hip arthroplasty. Arch Orthop Trauma Surg. 2006 Mar;126(2):134-7.

[89] Kop AM, Whitewood C, Johnston DJ. Damage of oxinium femoral heads subsequent to hip arthroplasty dislocation three retrieval case studies. J Arthroplasty. 2007 Aug; 22(5):775-9.

[90] McConway J, O'Brien S, Doran E, Archbold P, Beverland D. The use of a posterior lip augmentation device for a revision of recurrent dislocation after primary cemented Charnley/Charnley Elite total hip replacement: results at a mean follow-up of six years and nine months. J Bone Joint Surg Br. 2007 Dec;89(12):1581-5.

[91] Hofmann AA, Skrzynski MC. Leg-length inequality and nerve palsy in total hip arthroplasty: a lawyer awaits! Orthopedics. 2000 Sep;23(9):943-4.

[92] Konyves A, Bannister GC. The importance of leg length discrepancy after total hip arthroplasty. J Bone Joint Surg Br. 2005 Feb;87(2):155-7.

[93] Edwards BN, Tullos HS, Noble PC. Contributory factors and etiology of sciatic nerve palsy in total hip arthroplasty. Clin Orthop Relat Res. 1987 May(218):136-41.

[94] Farrell CM, Springer BD, Haidukewych GJ, Morrey BF. Motor nerve palsy following primary total hip arthroplasty. J Bone Joint Surg Am. 2005 Dec;87(12):2619-25.

[95] Gurney B, Mermier C, Robergs R, Gibson A, Rivero D. Effects of limb-length discrep-
      ancy on gait economy and lower-extremity muscle activity in older adults. J Bone
      Joint Surg Am. 2001 Jun;83-A(6):907-15.

[96] Maloney WJ, Keeney JA. Leg length discrepancy after total hip arthroplasty. J Ar-
      throplasty. 2004 Jun;19(4 Suppl 1):108-10.

[97] Desai AS, Connors L, Board TN. Functional and radiological evaluation of a simple
      intra operative technique to avoid limb length discrepancy in total hip arthroplasty.
      Hip Int. 2011 Apr 5;21(2):192-8.

[98] Mihalko WM, Phillips MJ, Krackow KA. Acute sciatic and femoral neuritis following
      total hip arthroplasty. A case report. J Bone Joint Surg Am. 2001 Apr;83-A(4):589-92.

[99] Shiramizu K, Naito M, Shitama T, Nakamura Y, Shitama H. L-shaped caliper for
      limb length measurement during total hip arthroplasty. J Bone Joint Surg Br. 2004
      Sep;86(7):966-9.

[100] Clark CR, Huddleston HD, Schoch EP, 3rd, Thomas BJ. Leg-length discrepancy after
      total hip arthroplasty. J Am Acad Orthop Surg. 2006 Jan;14(1):38-45.

[101] Charnley J. A Clean-Air Operating Enclosure. Br J Surg. 1964 Mar;51:202-5.

[102] Lister J. Antiseptic principle in the practice of surgery. Br Med J. 1967 Apr 1;2(5543):
      9-12.

[103] Charnley J. Low Friction Arthroplasty of the Hip Theory and Practice. Berlin/Heidel-
      berg: Springer-Verlag; 1979.

[104] Lidwell OM, Lowbury EJ, Whyte W, Blowers R, Stanley SJ, Lowe D. Effect of ultra-
      clean air in operating rooms on deep sepsis in the joint after total hip or knee replace-
      ment: a randomised study. Br Med J (Clin Res Ed). 1982 Jul 3;285(6334):10-4.

[105] Bannister G. (v) Prevention of infection in joint replacement. Current Orthopaedics.
      2002;16(6):426-33.

[106] Ericson C, Lidgren L, Lindberg L. Cloxacillin in the prophylaxis of postoperative in-
      fections of the hip. J Bone Joint Surg Am. 1973 Jun;55(4):808-13, 43.

[107] Nelson CL, Green TG, Porter RA, Warren RD. One day versus seven days of preven-
      tive antibiotic therapy in orthopedic surgery. Clin Orthop Relat Res. 1983 Jun(176):
      258-63.

[108] Charnley J, Eftekhar N. Postoperative infection in total prosthetic replacement ar-
      throplasty of the hip-joint. With special reference to the bacterial content of the air of
      the operating room. Br J Surg. 1969 Sep;56(9):641-9.

[109] Gambhir AK, Wroblewski BM, Kay PR. (iii) The infected total hip replacement. Cur-
      rent Orthopaedics. 2000;14(4):257-61.

[110] Pulido L, Ghanem E, Joshi A, Purtill JJ, Parvizi J. Periprosthetic joint infection: the incidence, timing, and predisposing factors. Clin Orthop Relat Res. 2008 Jul;466(7): 1710-5.

[111] Dunne WM, Jr. Bacterial adhesion: seen any good biofilms lately? Clin Microbiol Rev. 2002 Apr;15(2):155-66.

[112] Gristina AG, Shibata Y, Giridhar G, Kreger A, Myrvik QN. The glycocalyx, biofilm, microbes, and resistant infection. Semin Arthroplasty. 1994 Oct;5(4):160-70.

[113] Tsukayama DT, Estrada R, Gustilo RB. Infection after total hip arthroplasty. A study of the treatment of one hundred and six infections. J Bone Joint Surg Am. 1996 Apr; 78(4):512-23.

[114] Levitsky KA, Hozack WJ, Balderston RA, Rothman RH, Gluckman SJ, Maslack MM, et al. Evaluation of the painful prosthetic joint. Relative value of bone scan, sedimentation rate, and joint aspiration. J Arthroplasty. 1991 Sep;6(3):237-44.

[115] Kraemer WJ, Saplys R, Waddell JP, Morton J. Bone scan, gallium scan, and hip aspiration in the diagnosis of infected total hip arthroplasty. J Arthroplasty. 1993 Dec; 8(6):611-6.

[116] Bauer TW, Parvizi J, Kobayashi N, Krebs V. Diagnosis of periprosthetic infection. J Bone Joint Surg Am. 2006 Apr;88(4):869-82.

[117] Zhuang H, Yang H, Alavi A. Critical role of 18F-labeled fluorodeoxyglucose PET in the management of patients with arthroplasty. Radiol Clin North Am. 2007 Jul;45(4): 711-8, vii.

[118] Love C, Marwin SE, Palestro CJ. Nuclear medicine and the infected joint replacement. Semin Nucl Med. 2009 Jan;39(1):66-78.

[119] Spangehl MJ, Masri BA, O'Connell JX, Duncan CP. Prospective analysis of preoperative and intraoperative investigations for the diagnosis of infection at the sites of two hundred and two revision total hip arthroplasties. J Bone Joint Surg Am. 1999 May; 81(5):672-83.

[120] Di Cesare PE, Chang E, Preston CF, Liu CJ. Serum interleukin-6 as a marker of periprosthetic infection following total hip and knee arthroplasty. J Bone Joint Surg Am. 2005 Sep;87(9):1921-7.

[121] Crockarell JR, Hanssen AD, Osmon DR, Morrey BF. Treatment of infection with debridement and retention of the components following hip arthroplasty. J Bone Joint Surg Am. 1998 Sep;80(9):1306-13.

[122] Buchholz HW, Elson RA, Engelbrecht E, Lodenkamper H, Rottger J, Siegel A. Management of deep infection of total hip replacement. J Bone Joint Surg Br. 1981;63-B(3): 342-53.

[123] Jackson WO, Schmalzried TP. Limited role of direct exchange arthroplasty in the treatment of infected total hip replacements. Clin Orthop Relat Res. 2000 Dec(381): 101-5.

[124] Younger AS, Duncan CP, Masri BA, McGraw RW. The outcome of two-stage arthroplasty using a custom-made interval spacer to treat the infected hip. J Arthroplasty. 1997 Sep;12(6):615-23.

[125] Stockley I, Mockford BJ, Hoad-Reddick A, Norman P. The use of two-stage exchange arthroplasty with depot antibiotics in the absence of long-term antibiotic therapy in infected total hip replacement. J Bone Joint Surg Br. 2008 Feb;90(2):145-8.

[126] Sanchez-Sotelo J, Berry DJ, Hanssen AD, Cabanela ME. Midterm to long-term follow-up of staged reimplantation for infected hip arthroplasty. Clin Orthop Relat Res. 2009 Jan;467(1):219-24.

[127] Haddad FS, Masri BA, Garbuz DS, Duncan CP. The treatment of the infected hip replacement. The complex case. Clin Orthop Relat Res. 1999 Dec(369):144-56.

[128] McDonald DJ, Fitzgerald RH, Jr., Ilstrup DM. Two-stage reconstruction of a total hip arthroplasty because of infection. J Bone Joint Surg Am. 1989 Jul;71(6):828-34.

[129] Schmalzried TP, Noordin S, Amstutz HC. Update on nerve palsy associated with total hip replacement. Clin Orthop Relat Res. 1997 Nov(344):188-206.

[130] Barrack RL. Neurovascular injury: avoiding catastrophe. J Arthroplasty. 2004 Jun; 19(4 Suppl 1):104-7.

[131] Schmalzried T, Amstutz H, Dorey F. Nerve palsy associated with total hip replacement. Risk factors and prognosis. J Bone Joint Surg Am. 1991 August 1, 1991;73(7): 1074-80.

[132] Jolles BM, Bogoch ER. Posterior versus lateral surgical approach for total hip arthroplasty in adults with osteoarthritis. Cochrane Database Syst Rev. 2006;3:CD003828.

[133] Yuen EC, Olney RK, So YT. Sciatic neuropathy: clinical and prognostic features in 73 patients. Neurology. 1994 Sep;44(9):1669-74.

[134] Calligaro KD, Dougherty MJ, Ryan S, Booth RE. Acute arterial complications associated with total hip and knee arthroplasty. J Vasc Surg. 2003 Dec;38(6):1170-7.

[135] Abularrage CJ, Weiswasser JM, Dezee KJ, Slidell MB, Henderson WG, Sidawy AN. Predictors of lower extremity arterial injury after total knee or total hip arthroplasty. J Vasc Surg. 2008 Apr;47(4):803-7; discussion 7-8.

[136] Parvizi J, Pulido L, Slenker N, Macgibeny M, Purtill JJ, Rothman RH. Vascular injuries after total joint arthroplasty. J Arthroplasty. 2008 Dec;23(8):1115-21.

[137] Wilson JS, Miranda A, Johnson BL, Shames ML, Back MR, Bandyk DF. Vascular injuries associated with elective orthopedic procedures. Ann Vasc Surg. 2003 Nov;17(6): 641-4.

[138] Doi S, Motoyama Y, Itoh H. External iliac vein injury during total hip arthroplasty resulting in delayed shock. Br J Anaesth. 2005 Jun;94(6):866.

[139] Wasielewski RC, Crossett LS, Rubash HE. Neural and vascular injury in total hip arthroplasty. Orthop Clin North Am. 1992 Apr;23(2):219-35.

[140] Malchau H, Herberts P, Eisler T, Garellick G, Soderman P. The Swedish Total Hip Replacement Register. J Bone Joint Surg Am. 2002;84-A Suppl 2:2-20.

[141] Willert HG. Reactions of the articular capsule to wear products of artificial joint prostheses. J Biomed Mater Res. 1977 Mar;11(2):157-64.

[142] Maloney WJ, Smith RL. Periprosthetic osteolysis in total hip arthroplasty: the role of particulate wear debris. Instr Course Lect. 1996;45:171-82.

[143] Holt G, Murnaghan C, Reilly J, Meek RM. The biology of aseptic osteolysis. Clin Orthop Relat Res. 2007 Jul;460:240-52.

[144] Hirakawa K, Jacobs JJ, Urban R, Saito T. Mechanisms of failure of total hip replacements: lessons learned from retrieval studies. Clin Orthop Relat Res. 2004 Mar(420): 10-7.

[145] Aspenberg P, Van der Vis H. Migration, particles, and fluid pressure. A discussion of causes of prosthetic loosening. Clin Orthop Relat Res. 1998 Jul(352):75-80.

[146] van der Vis H, Aspenberg P, de Kleine R, Tigchelaar W, van Noorden CJ. Short periods of oscillating fluid pressure directed at a titanium-bone interface in rabbits lead to bone lysis. Acta Orthop Scand. 1998 Feb;69(1):5-10.

[147] Walter WL, Walter WK, O'Sullivan M. The pumping of fluid in cementless cups with holes. J Arthroplasty. 2004 Feb;19(2):230-4.

[148] Robertsson O, Wingstrand H, Kesteris U, Jonsson K, Onnerfalt R. Intracapsular pressure and loosening of hip prostheses. Preoperative measurements in 18 hips. Acta Orthop Scand. 1997 Jun;68(3):231-4.

[149] Abu-Amer Y, Darwech I, Clohisy JC. Aseptic loosening of total joint replacements: mechanisms underlying osteolysis and potential therapies. Arthritis Res Ther. 2007;9 Suppl 1:S6.

[150] Purdue PE, Koulouvaris P, Potter HG, Nestor BJ, Sculco TP. The cellular and molecular biology of periprosthetic osteolysis. Clin Orthop Relat Res. 2007 Jan;454:251-61.

[151] Goldring S, Schiller A, Roelke M, Rourke C, O'Neil D, Harris W. The synovial-like membrane at the bone-cement interface in loose total hip replacements and its proposed role in bone lysis. J Bone Joint Surg Am. 1983 June 1, 1983;65(5):575-84.

[152] Malik MH, Bayat A, Jury F, Ollier WE, Kay PR. Genetic susceptibility to hip arthroplasty failure--association with the RANK/OPG pathway. Int Orthop. 2006 Jun;30(3): 177-81.

[153] Malik MH, Jury F, Bayat A, Ollier WE, Kay PR. Genetic susceptibility to total hip arthroplasty failure: a preliminary study on the influence of matrix metalloproteinase 1, interleukin 6 polymorphisms and vitamin D receptor. Ann Rheum Dis. 2007 Aug; 66(8):1116-20.

[154] Gordon A, Kiss-Toth E, Stockley I, Eastell R, Wilkinson JM. Polymorphisms in the interleukin-1 receptor antagonist and interleukin-6 genes affect risk of osteolysis in patients with total hip arthroplasty. Arthritis Rheum. 2008 Oct;58(10):3157-65.

[155] Wilkinson JM, Wilson AG, Stockley I, Scott IR, Macdonald DA, Hamer AJ, et al. Variation in the TNF gene promoter and risk of osteolysis after total hip arthroplasty. J Bone Miner Res. 2003 Nov;18(11):1995-2001.

[156] Engh CA, Jr., Stepniewski AS, Ginn SD, Beykirch SE, Sychterz-Terefenko CJ, Hopper RH, Jr., et al. A randomized prospective evaluation of outcomes after total hip arthroplasty using cross-linked marathon and non-cross-linked Enduron polyethylene liners. J Arthroplasty. 2006 Sep;21(6 Suppl 2):17-25.

[157] Muratoglu OK, Bragdon CR, O'Connor DO, Jasty M, Harris WH. A novel method of cross-linking ultra-high-molecular-weight polyethylene to improve wear, reduce oxidation, and retain mechanical properties. Recipient of the 1999 HAP Paul Award. J Arthroplasty. 2001 Feb;16(2):149-60.

[158] Lusty PJ, Tai CC, Sew-Hoy RP, Walter WL, Walter WK, Zicat BA. Third-generation alumina-on-alumina ceramic bearings in cementless total hip arthroplasty. J Bone Joint Surg Am. 2007 Dec;89(12):2676-83.

[159] Lusty PJ, Watson A, Tuke MA, Walter WL, Walter WK, Zicat B. Wear and acetabular component orientation in third generation alumina-on-alumina ceramic bearings: an analysis of 33 retrievals [corrected]. J Bone Joint Surg Br. 2007 Sep;89(9):1158-64.

[160] Smith SL, Unsworth A. An in vitro wear study of alumina-alumina total hip prostheses. Proc Inst Mech Eng [H]. 2001;215(5):443-6.

[161] Clarke IC, Good V, Williams P, Schroeder D, Anissian L, Stark A, et al. Ultra-low wear rates for rigid-on-rigid bearings in total hip replacements. Proc Inst Mech Eng [H]. 2000;214(4):331-47.

[162] Fisher J, Jin Z, Tipper J, Stone M, Ingham E. Tribology of alternative bearings. Clin Orthop Relat Res. 2006 Dec;453:25-34.

[163] McKellop H, Park SH, Chiesa R, Doorn P, Lu B, Normand P, et al. In vivo wear of three types of metal on metal hip prostheses during two decades of use. Clin Orthop Relat Res. 1996 Aug(329 Suppl):S128-40.

[164] Streicher RM, Semlitsch M, Schon R, Weber H, Rieker C. Metal-on-metal articulation for artificial hip joints: laboratory study and clinical results. Proc Inst Mech Eng [H]. 1996;210(3):223-32.

[165] Illgen RL, 2nd, Bauer LM, Hotujec BT, Kolpin SE, Bakhtiar A, Forsythe TM. Highly crosslinked vs conventional polyethylene particles: relative in vivo inflammatory response. J Arthroplasty. 2009 Jan;24(1):117-24.

[166] Illgen RL, 2nd, Forsythe TM, Pike JW, Laurent MP, Blanchard CR. Highly cross-linked vs conventional polyethylene particles--an in vitro comparison of biologic activities. J Arthroplasty. 2008 Aug;23(5):721-31.

[167] Khan NQ, Woolson ST. Referral patterns of hip pain in patients undergoing total hip replacement. Orthopedics. 1998 Feb;21(2):123-6.

[168] Shih LY, Wu JJ, Yang DJ. Erythrocyte sedimentation rate and C-reactive protein values in patients with total hip arthroplasty. Clin Orthop Relat Res. 1987 Dec(225): 238-46.

[169] Temmerman OP, Raijmakers PG, Berkhof J, Hoekstra OS, Teule GJ, Heyligers IC. Accuracy of diagnostic imaging techniques in the diagnosis of aseptic loosening of the femoral component of a hip prosthesis: a meta-analysis. J Bone Joint Surg Br. 2005 Jun;87(6):781-5.

[170] Walde TA, Weiland DE, Leung SB, Kitamura N, Sychterz CJ, Engh CA, Jr., et al. Comparison of CT, MRI, and radiographs in assessing pelvic osteolysis: a cadaveric study. Clin Orthop Relat Res. 2005 Aug(437):138-44.

[171] Leung S, Naudie D, Kitamura N, Walde T, Engh CA. Computed tomography in the assessment of periacetabular osteolysis. J Bone Joint Surg Am. 2005 Mar;87(3):592-7.

[172] Talmo CT, Shanbhag AS, Rubash HE. Nonsurgical management of osteolysis: challenges and opportunities. Clin Orthop Relat Res. 2006 Dec;453:254-64.

[173] Stulberg BN, Della Valle AG. What are the guidelines for the surgical and nonsurgical treatment of periprosthetic osteolysis? J Am Acad Orthop Surg. 2008;16 Suppl 1:S20-5.

[174] Squire M, Griffin WL, Mason JB, Peindl RD, Odum S. Acetabular component deformation with press-fit fixation. J Arthroplasty. 2006 Sep;21(6 Suppl 2):72-7.

[175] Langdown AJ, Pickard RJ, Hobbs CM, Clarke HJ, Dalton DJ, Grover ML. Incomplete seating of the liner with the Trident acetabular system: a cause for concern? J Bone Joint Surg Br. 2007 Mar;89(3):291-5.

[176] Tateiwa T, Clarke IC, Williams PA, Garino J, Manaka M, Shishido T, et al. Ceramic total hip arthroplasty in the United States: safety and risk issues revisited. Am J Orthop. 2008 Feb;37(2):E26-31.

[177] D'Antonio JA, Capello WN, Manley MT, Naughton M, Sutton K. A titanium-encased alumina ceramic bearing for total hip arthroplasty: 3- to 5-year results. Clin Orthop Relat Res. 2005 Dec;441:151-8.

[178] Willmann G. Ceramic femoral head retrieval data. Clin Orthop Relat Res. 2000 Oct(379):22-8.

[179] Ha YC, Kim SY, Kim HJ, Yoo JJ, Koo KH. Ceramic liner fracture after cementless alumina-on-alumina total hip arthroplasty. Clin Orthop Relat Res. 2007 May;458:106-10.

[180] Koo KH, Ha YC, Jung WH, Kim SR, Yoo JJ, Kim HJ. Isolated fracture of the ceramic head after third-generation alumina-on-alumina total hip arthroplasty. J Bone Joint Surg Am. 2008 Feb;90(2):329-36.

[181] Weisse B, Affolter C, Stutz A, Terrasi GP, Kobel S, Weber W. Influence of contaminants in the stem-ball interface on the static fracture load of ceramic hip joint ball heads. Proc Inst Mech Eng [H]. 2008 Jul;222(5):829-35.

[182] Min BW, Song KS, Kang CH, Bae KC, Won YY, Lee KY. Delayed fracture of a ceramic insert with modern ceramic total hip replacement. J Arthroplasty. 2007 Jan;22(1): 136-9.

[183] Restrepo C, Parvizi J, Kurtz SM, Sharkey PF, Hozack WJ, Rothman RH. The noisy ceramic hip: is component malpositioning the cause? J Arthroplasty. 2008 Aug;23(5): 643-9.

[184] Keurentjes JC, Kuipers RM, Wever DJ, Schreurs BW. High incidence of squeaking in THAs with alumina ceramic-on-ceramic bearings. Clin Orthop Relat Res. 2008 Jun; 466(6):1438-43.

[185] Walter WL, Insley GM, Walter WK, Tuke MA. Edge loading in third generation alumina ceramic-on-ceramic bearings: stripe wear. J Arthroplasty. 2004 Jun;19(4):402-13.

[186] Taylor S, Manley MT, Sutton K. The role of stripe wear in causing acoustic emissions from alumina ceramic-on-ceramic bearings. J Arthroplasty. 2007 Oct;22(7 Suppl 3): 47-51.

[187] Manley MT, Sutton K. Bearings of the future for total hip arthroplasty. J Arthroplasty. 2008 Oct;23(7 Suppl):47-50.

[188] Doorn PF, Campbell PA, Worrall J, Benya PD, McKellop HA, Amstutz HC. Metal wear particle characterization from metal on metal total hip replacements: transmission electron microscopy study of periprosthetic tissues and isolated particles. J Biomed Mater Res. 1998 Oct;42(1):103-11.

[189] Daniel J, Ziaee H, Pradhan C, McMinn DJ. Six-year results of a prospective study of metal ion levels in young patients with metal-on-metal hip resurfacings. J Bone Joint Surg Br. 2009 Feb;91(2):176-9.

[190] De Smet K, De Haan R, Calistri A, Campbell PA, Ebramzadeh E, Pattyn C, et al. Metal ion measurement as a diagnostic tool to identify problems with metal-on-metal hip resurfacing. J Bone Joint Surg Am. 2008 Nov;90 Suppl 4:202-8.

[191] De Haan R, Pattyn C, Gill HS, Murray DW, Campbell PA, De Smet K. Correlation between inclination of the acetabular component and metal ion levels in metal-on-metal hip resurfacing replacement. J Bone Joint Surg Br. 2008 Oct;90(10):1291-7.

[192] Savarino L, Padovani G, Ferretti M, Greco M, Cenni E, Perrone G, et al. Serum ion levels after ceramic-on-ceramic and metal-on-metal total hip arthroplasty: 8-year minimum follow-up. J Orthop Res. 2008 Dec;26(12):1569-76.

[193] MacDonald SJ. Can a safe level for metal ions in patients with metal-on-metal total hip arthroplasties be determined? J Arthroplasty. 2004 Dec;19(8 Suppl 3):71-7.

[194] Keegan GM, Learmonth ID, Case CP. Orthopaedic metals and their potential toxicity in the arthroplasty patient: A review of current knowledge and future strategies. J Bone Joint Surg Br. 2007 May;89(5):567-73.

[195] Hart AJ, Hester T, Sinclair K, Powell JJ, Goodship AE, Pele L, et al. The association between metal ions from hip resurfacing and reduced T-cell counts. J Bone Joint Surg Br. 2006 Apr;88(4):449-54.

[196] Ziaee H, Daniel J, Datta AK, Blunt S, McMinn DJ. Transplacental transfer of cobalt and chromium in patients with metal-on-metal hip arthroplasty: a controlled study. J Bone Joint Surg Br. 2007 Mar;89(3):301-5.

[197] Keegan GM, Learmonth ID, Case CP. A systematic comparison of the actual, potential, and theoretical health effects of cobalt and chromium exposures from industry and surgical implants. Crit Rev Toxicol. 2008;38(8):645-74.

[198] Smith AJ, Dieppe P, Porter M, Blom AW. Risk of cancer in first seven years after metal-on-metal hip replacement compared with other bearings and general population: linkage study between the National Joint Registry of England and Wales and hospital episode statistics. BMJ. 2012;344:e2383.

[199] Hart AJ, Buddhdev P, Winship P, Faria N, Powell JJ, Skinner JA. Cup inclination angle of greater than 50 degrees increases whole blood concentrations of cobalt and chromium ions after metal-on-metal hip resurfacing. Hip Int. 2008 Jul-Sep;18(3):212-9.

[200] Willert HG, Buchhorn GH, Fayyazi A, Flury R, Windler M, Koster G, et al. Metal-on-metal bearings and hypersensitivity in patients with artificial hip joints. A clinical and histomorphological study. J Bone Joint Surg Am. 2005 Jan;87(1):28-36.

[201] Pandit H, Glyn-Jones S, McLardy-Smith P, Gundle R, Whitwell D, Gibbons CL, et al. Pseudotumours associated with metal-on-metal hip resurfacings. J Bone Joint Surg Br. 2008 Jul;90(7):847-51.

[202] Pandit H, Vlychou M, Whitwell D, Crook D, Luqmani R, Ostlere S, et al. Necrotic granulomatous pseudotumours in bilateral resurfacing hip arthoplasties: evidence for a type IV immune response. Virchows Arch. 2008 Nov;453(5):529-34.

[203] Haddad FS, Thakrar RR, Hart AJ, Skinner JA, Nargol AV, Nolan JF, et al. Metal-on-metal bearings: the evidence so far. J Bone Joint Surg Br. 2011 May;93(5):572-9.

[204] Smith AJ, Dieppe P, Vernon K, Porter M, Blom AW. Failure rates of stemmed metal-on-metal hip replacements: analysis of data from the National Joint Registry of England and Wales. Lancet. 2012 Mar 31;379(9822):1199-204.

[205] Fink B, Fuerst M, Singer J. Periprosthetic fractures of the femur associated with hip arthroplasty. Arch Orthop Trauma Surg. 2005 Sep;125(7):433-42.

[206] Duncan CP, Masri BA. Fractures of the femur after hip replacement. Instr Course Lect. 1995;44:293-304.

[207] McElfresh EC, Coventry MB. Femoral and pelvic fractures after total hip arthroplasty. J Bone Joint Surg Am. 1974 Apr;56(3):483-92.

[208] Haidukewych GJ, Jacofsky DJ, Hanssen AD, Lewallen DG. Intraoperative fractures of the acetabulum during primary total hip arthroplasty. J Bone Joint Surg Am. 2006 Sep;88(9):1952-6.

[209] Davidson D, Pike J, Garbuz D, Duncan CP, Masri BA. Intraoperative periprosthetic fractures during total hip arthroplasty. Evaluation and management. J Bone Joint Surg Am. 2008 Sep;90(9):2000-12.

[210] Sharkey PF, Hozack WJ, Callaghan JJ, Kim YS, Berry DJ, Hanssen AD, et al. Acetabular fracture associated with cementless acetabular component insertion: a report of 13 cases. J Arthroplasty. 1999 Jun;14(4):426-31.

[211] Masri BA, Meek RM, Duncan CP. Periprosthetic fractures evaluation and treatment. Clin Orthop Relat Res. 2004 Mar;(420):80-95.

[212] Orzel JA, Rudd TG, Nelp WB. Heterotopic bone formation (myositis ossificans) and lower-extremity swelling mimicking deep-venous disease. J Nucl Med. 1984 Oct; 25(10):1105-7.

[213] owsey J CM, Robins PR. Heterotopic ossification: theoretical consideration possible etiological factors, and a clinical review of total hip arthroplasty patients exhibiting this phenomenon. The hip: procs 5th Open Scientific Meeting of the Hip Society. 1977:201-21.

[214] Brooker AF, Bowerman JW, Robinson RA, Riley LH, Jr. Ectopic ossification following total hip replacement. Incidence and a method of classification. J Bone Joint Surg Am. 1973 Dec;55(8):1629-32.

[215] Naraghi FF, DeCoster TA, Moneim MS, Miller RA, Rivero D. Heterotopic ossification. Orthopedics. 1996 Feb;19(2):145-51.

[216] Shafritz AB, Shore EM, Gannon FH, Zasloff MA, Taub R, Muenke M, et al. Overexpression of an osteogenic morphogen in fibrodysplasia ossificans progressiva. N Engl J Med. 1996 Aug 22;335(8):555-61.

[217] Hannallah D, Peng H, Young B, Usas A, Gearhart B, Huard J. Retroviral delivery of Noggin inhibits the formation of heterotopic ossification induced by BMP-4, demin-

eralized bone matrix, and trauma in an animal model. J Bone Joint Surg Am. 2004 Jan;86-A(1):80-91.

[218] Harris WH. Clinical results using the Mueller-Charnley total hip prosthesis. Clin Orthop Relat Res. 1972 Jul-Aug;86:95-101.

[219] Chao ST, Lee SY, Borden LS, Joyce MJ, Krebs VE, Suh JH. External beam radiation helps prevent heterotopic bone formation in patients with a history of heterotopic ossification. J Arthroplasty. 2006 Aug;21(5):731-6.

[220] Cobb TK, Berry DJ, Wallrichs SL, Ilstrup DM, Morrey BF. Functional outcome of excision of heterotopic ossification after total hip arthroplasty. Clin Orthop Relat Res. 1999 Apr(361):131-9.

[221] Pellegrini VD, Jr., Evarts CM. Radiation prophylaxis of heterotopic bone formation following total hip arthroplasty: current status. Semin Arthroplasty. 1992 Jul;3(3): 156-66.

[222] Gregoritch SJ, Chadha M, Pelligrini VD, Rubin P, Kantorowitz DA. Randomized trial comparing preoperative versus postoperative irradiation for prevention of heterotopic ossification following prosthetic total hip replacement: preliminary results. Int J Radiat Oncol Biol Phys. 1994 Aug 30;30(1):55-62.

[223] Lo TC, Healy WL, Covall DJ, Dotter WE, Pfeifer BA, Torgerson WR, et al. Heterotopic bone formation after hip surgery: prevention with single-dose postoperative hip irradiation. Radiology. 1988 Sep;168(3):851-4.

Chapter 2

Imaging Patellar Complications After Knee Arthroplasty

Pietro Melloni, Maite Veintemillas, Anna Marin and
Rafael Valls

Additional information is available at the end of the chapter

1. Introduction

Knee arthroplasty, like hip replacement, is becoming increasingly common as the overall population begins to age. The survival rate of the knee implant is also increasing and is now similar to that of hip prostheses (85%-90% at 15 years).

Although complications in knee replacements have been widely reported and discussed, the literature contains few studies about patellar complications after total or partial knee arthroplasty.

Patellar complications after knee arthroplasty are infrequent but they can lead to unsatisfactory clinical outcome. Complications are often underestimated because the femoral component makes visualization of these lesions difficult. Evaluation must begin with a thorough history and physical examination. Laboratory tests and imaging studies can provide additional evidence to support a particular diagnosis.

The aim of this chapter is to describe and analyze complications affecting the patella in patients with total or partial knee arthroplasty and to illustrate some representative examples of the spectrum of findings on different imaging techniques, such as plain-film radiography and ultrasound (US), with the emphasis on plain-film findings.

Together with the clinical examination and follow-up, thorough plain-film and computed tomography (CT) studies should be done before and after the surgery. Later follow-up is directed toward identifying complications such as instability/dislocation, fracture, osteonecrosis, infection, erosion, impingement on the prosthesis, patellar or quadriceps tendon tear, and loosening or rupture of the patellar prosthetic button. One large study demonstrated that obtaining plain-film radiographs immediately after knee arthroplasty is not cost-effective. [1]

In the follow-up, plain-film radiographs usually suffice for the assessment of patellar complications and are helpful for guiding treatment. Some authors recommend a weight-bearing axial radiograph to better assess patellofemoral kinematics. [2-3] Although radiographs are the mainstay in evaluating loosening or infection, they are limited by their less than optimal sensitivity and specificity. [4]

In one study, the sensitivity and specificity of plain-film radiography compared to the findings at surgery were 77% and 90%, respectively, for detecting femoral component loosening, and 83% and 72%, respectively, for detecting tibial component loosening. [5] However, no specific studies about patellar prosthetic button complications are found in the literature.

In the past, the roles of CT and magnetic resonance imaging (MRI) in the assessment of joint prostheses were inconsequential due to image degradation by artifact. However, improvements in techniques and instrumentation have greatly improved the usefulness of CT and MRI in patients with joint replacements. Although no studies have addressed the routine use of these techniques for the follow-up of asymptomatic patients, some authors recommend CT to look for osteolysis in patients with painful knee prostheses with normal or equivocal radiographs and increased uptake on all three phases of a bone scan. [6] Another group of researchers [7]- [8] recommend multidetector CT in cases where osteolysis is likely, such as those with aseptic loosening and gross polyethylene wear. In patients with loosening, CT examination may also be useful to show the extent and width of lucent zones that may be less apparent on radiographs; in these cases, CT makes it possible to assess rotational alignment of components and to detect subtle or occult periprosthetic fractures of the patella. [9-10]

We use CT to assess component alignment and position as well as rotation of the patella with respect to the femur in patients with knee arthroplasty.

In patients with metallic knee prostheses, we use MRI for very specific indications, such as to evaluate the soft tissues surrounding the patella like the patellar and quadriceps tendons, Hoffa's fat pad, prepatellar subcutaneous tissue, and others. Although MRI is the technique of choice to evaluate the soft tissues [11], its use is seriously limited by drawbacks such as the high cost of acquiring, installing, and maintaining the equipment; magnetic susceptibility; the difficulties of working in a magnetic field; the large number of artifacts; long examination times that may require sedation; discomfort due to the noise inside the scanner; and possible claustrophobia. However, now nearly all implants are non-magnetizable and modern scanners allow images to be manipulated, so magnetic artifacts are no longer a problem. Thus, it could be argued that MRI will eventually supplant US; [12]; for example, MR may be helpful in detecting extracapsular spread of infection and abscess formation. [13]

2. Material and methods

Every year between 1998 and 2011, our hospital carried out more than 200 total knee replacements and 10 to 15 implantations of unicompartmental prostheses of the knee. In some knee replacement procedures, the patella was left intact, but in others patellar resurfacing was performed or a prosthetic button was implanted. When the patella is intervened, it is often resurfaced with high-density polyethylene, which may be metal backed.

We retrospectively reviewed 1400 consecutive examinations in patients treated with total or partial knee arthroplasty in the last two years; 54 (3.7%) patients (35 women and 19 men) presented patellar complications. Mean patient age was 74 years (range, 55-90 years). In some cases, patients had prostheses in both knees.

All patients were followed up immediately after surgery, at 6 months, and then yearly or when necessary, using anteroposterior, lateral, and axial (Merchant view) radiographs. Lateral and axial projections are better for visualizing and evaluating the evolution of the patella after knee replacement.

In certain cases according to the clinical symptoms, patients underwent US, especially to evaluate the morphological integrity of the patellar and quadriceps tendons and other soft-tissue structures around the patella.

3. Results

The patellar complications that we observed following total knee arthroplasty include instability/dislocation, fracture, osteonecrosis, infection, erosion, impingement on the prosthesis, patellar or quadriceps tendon tear, and loosening or rupture of the patellar prosthetic button. The mean interval from total knee replacement to patellar complication was 5 years and 9 months (range, 5 months-15 years).

3.1. Instability/dislocation (n=21)

Patellar instability (n=15) is the commonest complication after knee arthroplasty. In total knee arthroplasty, most complications related to the extensor mechanism are caused by patellar maltracking instability. [14] Patellar maltracking may result from component malpositioning and limb malalignment, excessive femoral component size, prosthetic design, inadequate patellar resection, or soft-tissue imbalance. [15] Patellofemoral instability likely results most frequently from internal malrotation of the femoral or tibial components. [16]

Malpositioning of femoral and tibial components may affect patellar alignment. Although the axial rotation of the femoral component can be determined using plain-film radiographs or MRI, CT is most commonly used for this purpose. [17] Excessive combined internal rotation of tibial and femoral components is associated with patellar complications. [18] Furthermore, one study [19] found the amount of excessive combined internal rotation was directly proportional to the severity of patellofemoral complications. The rotation of the femoral component can be assessed with relation to the transepicondylar axis, the Whiteside line, or the posterior femoral condyles. The femoral component should be parallel to the transepicondylar axis and the tibial component should be in about 18 degrees of internal rotation with relation to the tibial tubercle.

Careful radiographic follow-up should be considered when deep flexion is achieved in a knee with a patella baja after total knee arthroplasty (Figure 1). Patellar dislocation (n=6) is mainly due to direct trauma to the patella or to extensor mechanism rupture [20] (Figure 2).

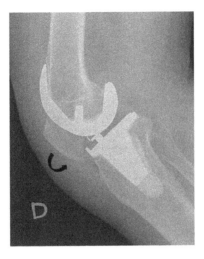

Figure 1. Patellar Instability. A 60-year-old man, five years after total knee replacement. Lateral radiograph reveals caudal displacement of the patella (curved arrow).

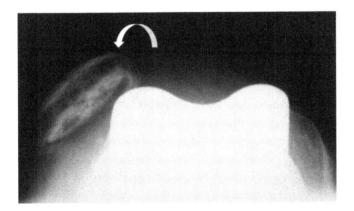

Figure 2. Patellar Dislocation. A 71-year-old woman, five years after total knee replacement. Axial radiograph (Merchant view) of the knee prosthesis with cemented prosthetic button of the patella demonstrates lateral patellar displacement on flexion (curved arrow).

Alterations in the patellotibial distance can occur during total knee arthroplasty due to excessive soft-tissue release that requires elevation of the joint to regain stability and placement of the polyethylene patellar component distally on the patella. Another cause of acquired patella baja seen commonly in total knee arthroplasty is elevation of the joint line, referred to as pseudo-patella baja. [21]

Radiographic evaluation of the patella primarily uses the lateral view and the sunrise or Merchant's view. This projection should show the central ridge of the patella lying at or medial to the bisector of the trochlear angle. This approach is also helpful for evaluating patellar tilt, but not it is very sensitive for determining the cause of patellofemoral pain.

The lateral view reveals the patellar thickness, inferior or superior positioning, as well as adequate fixation and position of the components. The positioning of the patellar component (centralized or tilted in relation to the trochlear sulcus or subluxated/dislocated) is clearly seen and may reveal the cause of instability. Tilt can be defined as medial or lateral, depending on its relation to the femoral condyles. Subluxation can be measured as displacement from the center of the prosthetic femoral intercondylar groove. [22]

3.2. Osteonecrosis (n=5)

Patellar resurfacing during total knee arthroplasty remains controversial. Several patellar complications such as fracture, avascular necrosis, and instability are related to resurfacing. On the other hand, some authors report lower re-operation rates and postoperative pain when the patella is resurfaced. Attention should be directed to the ultimate patellar thickness. Whether or not to resurface should be determined based on the exact initial thickness. A thicker patella is prone to instability, whereas a thinner patella is associated with higher complication rates. Patellar fragmentation and sclerosis of the fragments are presumed to represent osteonecrosis (Figure 3). The osteonecrosis may be due to disruption of the vascular network of the patella during total knee replacement surgery. [23] Medial parapatellar arthrotomy, fat pad removal, and lateral release all contribute to patellar devascularization. Evolutional osteonecrosis may lead to patellar fracture.

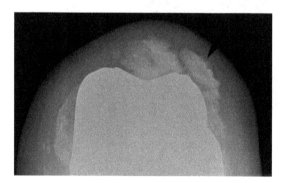

Figure 3. Patellar Necrosis. A 68-year-old man, seven years after total knee replacement. Axial radiograph of the knee prosthesis shows bony sclerosis with fragmentation of the patella (arrow).

3.3. Fracture (n=9)

Patellar fractures in association with total knee replacement are uncommon and occur predominantly in patients with resurfaced patellae. [24] Most fractures appear to occur in the first few years after total knee replacement.

Patient, implant, and technical factors are important predisposing causes of these patellar fractures. Avascularity, trauma, fatigue, and stress also play an etiologic role in some patellar fractures.

Trauma to the patella, either direct or indirect, and increased patellofemoral stress are other causes of fracture. Indirect causes might include an eccentric quadriceps muscle contraction associated with a stumble, resulting in an avulsion fracture (Figure 4).

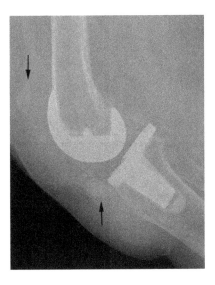

Figure 4. Patellar Avulsion Fracture. A 73-year-old woman, seven years after total knee replacement. Lateral radiograph shows a transverse avulsion fracture in the mid-portion of the patella with displacement of its poles in the cranial-caudal direction (arrows).

Patellar fractures are not associated with prior injury. Because patellar fractures are often asymptomatic and discovered incidentally, follow-up radiographs are essential for their detection. Transverse fractures seem to be related to patellar maltracking, and vertical fractures often occur through a fixation hole. CT or MRI can detect some fractures that go undetected on plain-film radiographs.

Prevention is the best treatment. Important outcome criteria include the integrity of the extensor mechanism, patellar implant fixation, and anatomic location. Surgery on patients with patella fractures has a high complication rate and should be avoided if possible. [25-26]

3.4. Infection (n=2)

Although rare, infection can appear in the patella after total or partial replacement of the knee. [27] Unspecific radiological signs of infection include a lytic lesion or osseous sclerosis in the patella or in the joint facet of the femur in the femoropatellar joint (Figure 5). Clinical symptoms may orient the diagnosis of infection.

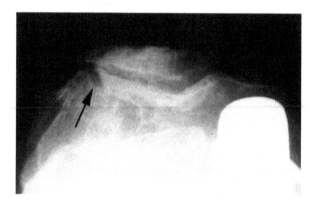

Figure 5. Patellar Infection. A 70-year-old man, nine years after partial knee replacement. Axial radiograph (Merchant view) of the knee prosthesis shows osteolysis on the lateral facet of the femur (arrow) with a non-cemented hemiarthroplasty of the knee, corresponding to a focus of infection, with sclerosis in the patella, suspected of infective infiltration. These findings were confirmed during surgery, and excisional debridement of the infection and total patellectomy were performed. Cultures were positive for *Pseudomonas aeruginosa*.

Plain-film radiographs are usually negative in the first ten days, even when clinical signs raise suspicion of infection. The radiological presentation varies, sometimes including localized rarefaction in the patella with or without sequestrum, or osseous destruction of the patella with or without an irregular bony fragment adjacent.

Surgical biopsy would provide the definitive diagnosis. The treatment of osteolytic lesions of the patella should be surgical.

3.5. Erosion/Impingement (n=6)

Patellar instability can cause erosion (n=2) in the joint facet of the patella due to friction with the femoral component of the knee arthroplasty (Figure 6). The erosion may appear as a lytic lesion that can simulate a subchondral cyst due to any arthritic process or small particle disease. Careful comparison with the pre-arthroplasty plain-films is essential. The erosion should not be confused with a dorsal defect in the posterior surface of the patella that occasionally persists into later life. The dorsal patellar defect is usually well delineated.

Patellar impingement (n=4), the so-called patellar clunk syndrome, results from the formation of a fibrous nodule over the proximal pole of the patella and reportedly occurs in cases of total kneed arthroplasty in which a posterior stabilized design is utilized. [28] Arthroscopic or open resection of the fibrous nodule can eliminate this syndrome.

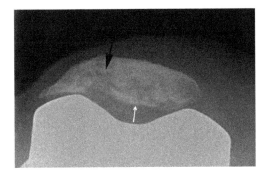

Figure 6. Patellar Osteolysis. A 75-year-old man, three years after total knee replacement. Axial radiograph (Merchant view) shows osteolysis of the lateral facet of the patella (black arrow) due to the loosening of both the total knee prosthesis and the patellar prosthetic button (white arrow). There was clinical suspicion of infection but cultures were negative.

Patellar impingement also is seen when patella baja develops after posterior stabilized total knee arthroplasty and when the patella becomes impinged against the femoral component (Figure 7). [29] Patellofemoral complications (osteoarthritis and impingement) are rarely seen after total replacement and even more rarely after unicompartmental arthroplasty [30], so their long-term consequences are not well known.

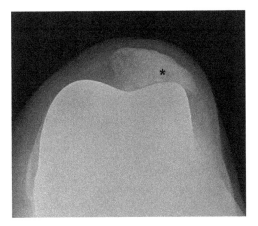

Figure 7. Patellar Impingement. A 71-year-old man, four years after total knee replacement. Axial radiograph (Merchant view) shows a reduction in the space between the knee arthroplasty and the patella, with consequent reactive patellar sclerosis (asterisk).

However, in our study the symptoms in knees with patellar impingement were usually more severe than in knees with degenerative changes.

3.7. Loosening or rupture of the patellar prosthetic button (n=7)

A patellar prosthetic button (patellar component) is added to total knee replacement in certain cases. Like all joint prostheses (such as hip, knee, and small joints), the patellar button may loosen or rupture with the same or similar characteristic radiological signs as in the other joints. Loosening of the patellar button (Figure 8) may cause significant anterior pain. Thin fixation pegs, maltracking, and trauma frequently induce component loosening. Revision of a failed patellar component is typically associated with a relatively high complication rate.

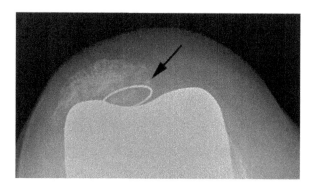

Figure 8. Prosthetic Button Loosening. A 71-year-old woman, two years after total knee replacement. Axial radiograph (Merchant view) shows patellar subluxation with prosthetic button loosening (arrow).

Osseous changes that may be observed in the patellar prosthetic button following total or partial knee arthroplasty include radiolucent lines, osteolysis, change in prosthesis position, and polyethylene wear. Radiolucent lines superimposed on the femoral component can often be obscured by the metal tray if the view is not perfectly tangential to the component surface. Nonprogressive focal radiolucent areas less than 2 mm in size are often insignificant; however, progressive, circumferential, radiolucent areas larger than 2 mm are often indicative of prosthesis loosening.

Rupture of the patellar prosthetic button (Figure 9) is rare but can occur due to polyethylene wear, fusion defects in the polyethylene structure [31], or trauma to the patella. [32] The incidence of wear in patients with all-polyethylene and metal-backed components ranges from 5% to 11%. Congruity, maltracking, and contact force are associated with polyethylene wear. Decreased polyethylene thickness in metal-backed designs is the determining factor for mechanism failure.

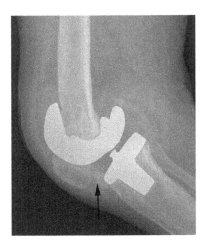

Figure 9. Prosthetic Button Rupture. A 68-year-old woman, four years after total knee replacement. Lateral radiograph shows a rupture of the patellar prosthetic button (arrow) with caudal displacement.

Prosthetic loosening, small particle disease, and infection are the most frequent causes of osteolysis of the patellar component. A change in position of components on serial images is indicative of prosthesis loosening. [33]

3.8. Patellar or quadriceps tendon tear (n=4)

Rupture of patellar or quadriceps ligaments occurs infrequently. However, the complications of an untreated rupture to the extensor mechanism can be extremely disabling. Contributing factors are excessive dissection and knee manipulation, and trauma. The same mechanical causes that produce patellar fractures can produce patellar [34] or quadriceps [35] tendon tear. US is the method of choice for studying the patellar or quadriceps tendons to confirm or rule out tendon tears (Figures 10 &11). An abrupt high patella is seen on lateral radiographs in some patients with clinical suspicion of tendon rupture after total knee replacement, but US is necessary to confirm the diagnosis. Although MRI can also be useful in this context, it is not widely used. Other diagnostic possibilities are chronic tendonitis or tendon laxness. Treatment outcomes for ruptured patellar ligaments are not good.

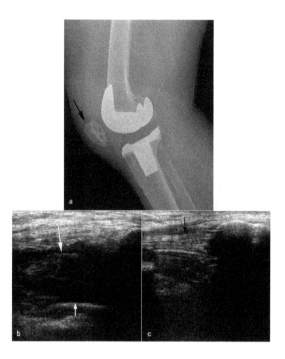

Figure 10. a-c).- **QuadricepsTendon Rupture.** A 73-year-old woman, ten years after total knee replacement. Lateral radiograph (a) shows patellar displacement and rotation with clinical suspicion of quadriceps tendon tear (black arrow). US (b) confirms a disrupted quadriceps tendon (long white arrow) with a suprapatellar fluid collection (short white arrow) and a 5 cm gap between the end of the tendon and the patella. Compare with the sonogram of the contralateral knee showing a normal quadriceps tendon (fine black arrow) with total knee replacement (c) in the same patient, who had rheumatoid arthritis.

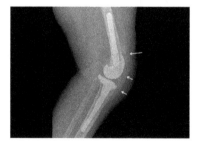

Figure 11. Patellar Tendon Rupture with Patellar Avulsion Fracture. A 69-year-old woman, twelve years after total knee replacement and two years after revision knee replacement with long femoral and tibial stems. Lateral radiograph shows cranial displacement with transverse avulsion fracture in the mid-portion of the patella (long arrow). Note the extensive soft-tissue edema in the patellar area (short arrows), leading to suspected patellar tendon rupture, which was confirmed at ultrasonography (not shown).

4. Conclusion

Patellar complications following knee arthroplasty are generally uncommon but often of potential clinical significance. Plain-film radiographs are essential for the evaluation of patellar complications after surgery and should be the initial imaging study performed. Careful attention to initial prosthesis placement and comparison of follow-up images will allow subtle abnormalities to be detected in patellar complications. US may have a special role in the evaluation of soft-tissue structures around the patella.

Author details

Pietro Melloni, Maite Veintemillas, Anna Marin and Rafael Valls

UDIAT Diagnostic Center, Corporació Sanitària i Universitària Parc Taulí, Sabadell, Spain

References

[1] Mendel E. Singer, PhD and Kimberly E. Applegate, MD. Cost-Effectiveness Analysis in Radiology. Departments of Epidemiology and Biostatistics, Metro Health Medical Center (M.E.S.), and the Department of Radiology, Rainbow Babies and Children's Hospital (K.E.A.), Case Western Reserve University School of Medicine, 10900 Euclid Ave, Cleveland, OH 44106 (M.E.S.)

[2] Nobuyuki Yoshino, Nobuyoshi Watanabe, Yukihisa Fukuda, Yoshinobu Watanabe, Shinro Takai. The influence of patellar dislocation on the femoro-tibial loading during total knee arthroplasty. Knee Surgery, Sports Traumatology, Arthroscopy. November 2011, Volume 19, Issue 11, pp 1817-1822.

[3] Shinro Takai, Nobuyuki Yoshino, Nobuyoshi Watanabe and Yukihisa Fukuda. The effect of patellar eversion to the extension and flexion gaps in total knee arthroplasty. J Bone Joint Surg Br 2010 vol. 92-b no. supp i 160-161.

[4] ACR Appropriateness Criteria® imaging after total knee arthroplasty. Weissman BN, Shah N, Daffner RH, Bancroft L, Bennett DL, Blebea JS, Bruno MA, Fries IB, Hayes CW, Kransdorf MJ, Luchs JS, Morrison WB, Palestro CJ, Roberts CC, Stoller DW, Taljanovic MS, Tuite MJ, Ward RJ, Wise JN, Zoga AC, Expert Panel on Musculoskeletal Imaging. ACR Appropriateness Criteria® imaging after total knee arthroplasty. [online publication]. Reston (VA): American College of Radiology (ACR).

[5] Jonathan Baré, MD, Steven J. MacDonald, Robert B. Bourne, MD. Preoperative Evaluations in Revision Total Knee Arthroplasty. Clinical Orthopaedics and Related Research. Number 446, pp. 40–44© 2006 Lippincott Williams & Wilkins.

[6] Use of multi-detector computed tomography for the detection of periprosthetic osteolysis in total knee arthroplasty. Reish TG, Clarke HD, Scuderi GR, Math KR, Scott WN. J Knee Surg. 2006 Oct;19(4):259-64.

[7] Imaging of total knee arthroplasty. Math KR, Zaidi SF, Petchprapa C, Harwin SF. Semin Musculoskelet Radiol. 2006 Mar;10(1):47-63. Review.

[8] Imaging of knee arthroplasty. Miller TT. Eur J Radiol. 2005 May;54(2):164-77. Review.

[9] Can CT-based patient-matched instrumentation achieve consistent rotational alignment in knee arthroplasty? Tibesku CO, Innocenti B, Wong P, Salehi A, Labey L. Arch Orthop Trauma Surg. 2012 Feb;132(2):171-7. Epub 2011 Oct 18.

[10] Rotational positioning of the tibial tray in total knee arthroplasty: a CT evaluation. Berhouet J, Beaufils P, Boisrenoult P, Frasca D, Pujol N. Orthop Traumatol Surg Res. 2011 Nov;97(7):699-704. Epub 2011 Oct 10.

[11] Magnetic resonance imaging of joint arthroplasty. Potter HG, Foo LF. Orthop Clin North Am. 2006 Jul;37(3):361-73, vi-vii. Review.

[12] Magnetic resonance imaging with metal suppression for evaluation of periprosthetic osteolysis after total knee arthroplasty. Vessely MB, Frick MA, Oakes D, Wenger DE, Berry DJ. J Arthroplasty. 2006 Sep;21(6):826-31.

[13] New MR imaging methods for metallic implants in the knee: artifact correction and clinical impact. Chen CA, Chen W, Goodman SB, Hargreaves BA, Koch KM, Lu W, Brau AC, Draper CE, Delp SL, Gold GE. J Magn Reson Imaging. 2011 May;33(5): 1121-7.

[14] Malo M, Vince KG. The unstable patella after total knee arthroplasty: etiology, prevention, and management. J Am Acad Orthop Surg. 2003 Sep-Oct;11(5):364-71.

[15] Robert Wen-Wei Hsu. The management of the patella in total knee arthroplasty. Chang Gung Med J. 2006 September-October. Vol. 29 No. 5.

[16] Efstathios K Motsis, Nikolaos Paschos, Emilios E Pakos, Anastasios D Georgoulis. Review article: Patellar instability after total knee arthroplasty. Journal of Orthopaedic Surgery 2009;17(3):351-7.

[17] Berger RA, Crossett LS, Jacobs JJ, Rubash HE; Malrotation causing patellofemoral complications after total knee arthroplasty. Clinical Orthopedics and Related Research. 1998 Nov;(356):144-53.

[18] Vanbiervliet J, Bellemans J, Innocenti B, et al. The influence of malrotation and femoral component material on patellofemoral wear during gait. Journal Of Bone & Joint Surgery, British Volume [serial online]. October 2011;93(10):1348-1354.

[19] Blisard R. Component internal rotation malrotation a factor in pain after TKA. Orthopedics Today [serial online]. September 2011;31(9):24.

[20] Rand JA. Extensor mechanism complications following total knee arthroplasty. J Knee Surg 2003;16:224–8.

[21] Chonko DJ, Lombardi AV Jr, Berend KR. Patella baja and total knee arthroplasty (TKA): etiology, diagnosis, and management. Surg Technol Int. 2004;12:231-8.

[22] Healy WL, Wasilewski SA, Takei R, Oberlander M. Patellofemoral complications following total knee arthroplasty. Correlation with implant design and patient risk factors. J Arthroplasty 1995;10:197–201.

[23] Kyung Ah, Chun Kenjirou, Ohashi D, Lee Bennett, Georges Y, El-Khoury. Patellar Fractures After Total Knee Replacement. AJR AM J Roent. 2005; sept, 185:655–660.

[24] Aglietti P, Baldini A, Buzzi R, Indelli PF. Patella resurfacing in total knee replacement: functional evaluation and complications. J Bone Joint Surg Am. 2002 Jul;84-A(7):1132-7.

[25] Bourne RB. Fractures of the patella after total knee replacement. Orthop Clin North AM. 1999 Apr; 30(2):287-91.

[26] Ortiguera CJ, Berry DJ. Patellar fracture after total knee arthroplasty. J Bone Joint Surg Am. 2002 Apr;84-A(4):532-40.

[27] Keating EM, Haas G, Meding JB. Patella fracture after total knee replacements. Clin Orthop. 2003 Nov;(416):93-7.

[28] Beight JL, Yao B, Hozack WJ, Hearn SL, Booth RE Jr. The patellar "clunk" syndrome after posterior stabilized total knee arthroplasty. Clin Orthop Relat Res. 1994 Feb; (299):139-42.

[29] Maeno S, Kondo M, Niki Y, Matsumoto H. Patellar impingement against the tibial component after total knee arthroplasty. Clin Orthop Relat Res. 2006. Nov; 452: 265.

[30] Matthew B. Collier, MS, et al. Osteolysis After Total Knee Arthroplasty: Influence of Tibial Baseplate Surface Finish and Sterilation of Polyethylene Insert. In The Journal of Bone and Joint Surgery. December 2005. Vol. 87-A. No. 12. Pp. 2702-2708.

[31] Hernigou P, Deschamps G. Patellar impingement following unicompartmental arthroplasty. J Bone Joint Surg Am. 2002 Jul;84-A(7):1132-7.

[32] MacCollum MS 3rd, Karpman RR. Complications of the PCA anatomic patella. Orthopedics. 1989 Nov;12(11):1423-8.

[33] William H Harris. Osteolysis and particle disease in hip replacement. A review. Acta Ortho~Scand 1994:65 113-123.

[34] Rand JA, Morrey BF, Bryan RS. Patellar tendon rupture after total knee arthroplasty. Clin Orthop Relat Res. 1989 Jul;(244):233-8.

[35] Dobbs RE, Hanssen AD, Lewallen DG, Pagnano MW. Quadriceps tendon rupture after total knee arthroplasty. Prevalence, complications, and outcomes. Bone Joint Surg Am. 2005 Jan;87(1):37-45.

Chapter 3

Periprosthetic Femoral Fractures in Total Knee Arthroplasty

Vladan Stevanović, Zoran Vukašinović,
Zoran Baščarević, Branislav Starčević,
Dragana Matanović and Duško Spasovski

Additional information is available at the end of the chapter

1. Introduction

Total joint arthroplasty has greatly improved the treatment of knee arthrosis, but still is not without complications. Supracondylar fractures above total knee replacements are an uncommon complication (incidence 0,3% to 2.5%), occuring more frequently in patients older than 60 years with osteoporotic bone. The rate of these fractures is expected to increase in the future because of the growing number of total knee replacements and greater level of acitivity among elderly patients. The timing of such fractures has been reported to range from early in the postoperative period to more than a decade after surgery, with a mean of 2 to 4 years. During the past two decades authors were not agreed in the definition of periprosthetic supracondylar region: the lower 3 inches (7cm) of the femur [1]; 9 cm proximal to the knee joint line [2]; all fractures within 15 cm proximal to the knee joint line [3]. Generally, based on the older literature, supracondylar periprosthetic fractures were those within 15 cm of the joint line, or in the case of stemmed component, within 5 cm of the proximal end of the implant. Nevertheless, the most important is understanding that these fractures occur in regions of stress concentration adjacent to a prosthetic component, and that the presence of the prosthesis has a significant effect on fracture treatment. So, we suggest that fractures above total knee replacement should be considered supracondylar fractures if they extend within 7 cm of the prosthetic joint line or if they are within 2 cm of the femoral prosthetic flange.

The most commonly suggested predisposing factors for a periprosthetic femoral fracture after total knee arthroplasty are osteopenia, revision arthroplasty, rheumatoid arthritis, use of steroids, existing neurological disorders, misalignment of the components, and notching of the anterior femoral cortex. Different factors were found in the pathogenesis of the fracture: stress-shielding from the anterior flange of the femoral component, inadequate osseous remodeling due to postoperative hypovascularity, relative difference in elastic modulus between the implant-covered distal part of the femur and femoral cortex, endosteal ischemia from metal or bone cement, and osteolysis of the distal part of the femur secondary to polyethylene wear debris. The majority of these fractures results from a combination of axial and torsion loads. Most of them occur following minimal falls, while the rest of them are secondary to motor-vehicle accidents, seizers or closed manipulation of a stiff knee after total knee arthroplasty

2. Prevalence and pathogenesis

The prevalence of supracondylar femoral fracture in patients with total knee replacement ranges from 0.3 to 4.2%. Most of the patients who sustain fractures about a total knee arthroplasty are women, usually in their seventh decade of life. As with other supracondylar fractures in the elderly, periprosthetic fractures usually occurs after low energy trauma. Osteoporosis is often present as well, due to a number of factors including stress shielding because of a rigid implant, pharmacologic causes, hormonal influences and senility. An association with rheumatoid arthritis, especially when the patient is receiving oral corticosteroid treatment, has been noted. Neurologic disorders have also been involved in the occurrence of these fractures, due to either medication induced osteoporosis or gait disturbance. In addition, revision arthroplasty has been associated with an increased incidence of periprosthetic fractures, more commonly when constrained implants are used, as they transfer applied torque more directly to bone that is potentially already deficient. Notching of the anterior femoral cortex during total knee arthroplasty has been indicated as one factor contributing to these periprosthetic femoral fractures. The prevalence of inadvertent cortical notching of the femur during total knee arthroplasty has been reported to be as high as 27% and there are several studies performed to quantify the reduction in bending and torsion strength resulting from femoral notching in attempt to provide the clinician with useful information related to the postoperative management [5, 6]. Clearly, notching of the anterior femoral cortex is neither the only risk factor nor the principal risk factor for supracondylar femoral fracture after knee replacement. Of a total of 6470 total knee arthroplasties included in reports on this subject, only seventeen (0.26%) were complicated by a supracondylar femoral fracture associated with anterior notching compared with nearly three times as many fractures that occurred in the absence of notching [5]; biomechanical effects of femoral notching following total knee arthroplasty showed mean decrease in bending strength of 18% (8-31%) and mean reduction in torsion strength of 39.2% (19-73%) in cadaveric specimens [6]. Based on Wolff's law, distal part of the femur would strengthen after the operation as result of remodeling, thus reduction in femoral bone strength should primarily be expected in the immediate postoperative period. Therefore a clear recommendation should be given to the patients who sustain inadvertent notching that they should have additional protection in the early postoperative period, and to consider the use a femoral component with stem as a means to bypass the stress riser of the anterior cortical notch. Most important, authors believe that an anterior cortical notch should be considered as a contraindication for manipulation of the knee prosthesis in the early postoperative period [7, 8].

Anterior defects may be present without notching, such as in cases of cystic lesions of degenerative or rheumatoid origin near the proximal aspect of the anterior femoral flange. Adequate remodeling may not be possible after those cysts are filled with cement at the time of arthroplasty. These defects remain as permanent stress risers, which may predispose to fracture. Large anterior effects might be better managed during primary knee arthroplasty with bone grafting and protection of the distal femur with an intramedullary stem [9].

Another recently recognized factor leading to late supracondylar femoral fracture is the presence of a massive debris-related osteolytic defect in the distal femur; such defects have been reported in association with asymptomatic well-fixed cementless femoral component. Ankylosis of a total knee arthroplasty may also predispose a fracture by producing increased stress in the distal femoral metaphysis [10, 11].

3. Risk factors / etiology

Literature data show that patients with osteopenia are at greater risk to acquire supracondylar femoral fracture after total knee arthroplasty, followed by rheumatoid arthritis, corticosteroid treatment, female gender and older age [12,13,14]. Additional risk factors are: neurological disorders, a revision total knee replacement (TKR) and rotationally constrained implants that create increased torsion load transfer to bone [15] (Table1).

Osteopenia
Rheumatoid arthritis
Steroid use
Neurologic disorders
Revision TKR
Female gender
Seventh decade of life
Distal femoral osteolysis
Anterior femoral notching +/-

Table 1. Risk factors for supracondylar femoral fractures, in decreasing order

Clinical and biomechanical data on anterior notching of the distal femoral cortex confirm the increase of fracture risk, and theoretical mathematical analysis calculated that a three-millimeter notch results in a 30% reduction in torsion bone strength [9]. On the other hand, a series of 670 total knee prosthesis with 20% femurs with anterior notching of at 3 mm at least, and found only two supracondylar fractures [11]. Different fracture patterns are associated with notched and no notched femurs: notched femurs tend to have short oblique fractures originating from the notched cortex, whereas no notched femurs tend to have diaphyseal fractures.

Furthermore, there is a general feeling that the most significant risk factor causing supracondylar fracture is the increase in activity that elderly patients achieve after knee replacement, exposing them to a greater risk of slipping and falling.

4. Diagnostic algorithm

Patients with this type of injury usually provide a history of minor trauma, such as fall during ambulation. They usually present with pain and inability to bear weight. Since these are typically low energy injuries, major tissue swelling is uncommon. Unless marked displacement is present, deformity may not be apparent on examination.

A thorough evaluation includes careful physical examination, a review of the patient's medical history and adequate radiographic studies. The injured limb should be assessed for soft tissue integrity and neurovascular status. The location of previous skin incisions must also be noted.

A complete radiographic examination of a fracture about a total knee arthroplasty includes standard anteroposterior and lateral radiographs as well as long leg views of the involved limb; oblique images and tomography are also often useful (Table 2). The diagnostic evaluation must include a direct lateral view of the distal femur in order to guide subsequent treatment: the direct lateral view facilitates assessment of fracture displacement, while also revealing the bone available for fixation devices, the location of femoral lugs of posterior cruciate retaining components and the proximal extent of the central femoral recess in cases with posterior stabilized components. Radiographically, nondisplaced or minimally displaced fractures may be obscured by the femoral flange; it is important to identify nondisplaced fractures since displacement may occur later.

Fracture displacement and comminution

Axial limb alignment

Quality of bone stock

Location of the fracture relative to the prosthesis

Stability of the prosthesis

Table 2. Characteristics of radiography assessment

Review of prefracture radiographs can provide important data regarding baseline limb alignment, implant fixation and the presence of regions of osteolysis or polyethylene wear. The type and technical specifications of the implant and templates in place will influence the selection of fixation device if open reduction is necessary [16, 17].

The first step is to establish whether the implant is loose; if so even if the fracture is well aligned and heals, treatment that does not include revision will lead to poor result. Prefracture misalignment, osteolysis and polyethylene wear are important factors in the decision making process.

The second step in the treatment is to identify fracture displacement and to decide whether reduction is needed. Any alteration in limb axis resulting from fracture can result in altered loading of the prosthesis, which may in turn lead to enhanced wear and/or accelerated implant loosening. The third step is to determine the appropriate treatment for displaced fracture (Figure 1).

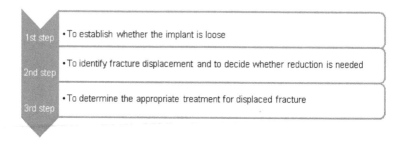

Figure 1. Diagnostic algorithm for periprosthetic supracondylar femoral fracture above total knee arthroplasty

5. Classification

Numerous systems of classification of supracondylar femoral fractures after total knee arthroplasty have been developed. Most of the classifications were based on supracondylar fractures without knee arthroplasty *(Neer et al, DiGioia and Rubash, Chen et al.)* (Table 3).

Neer et al.	Type I	Undisplaced (<5mm displacement or <5^0 angulation)*
	Type II	Displaced >1cm
	Type IIa	With lateral femoral shaft displacement
	Type IIb	With medial femoral shaft displacement
	Type III	Displaced and comminuted
DiGioia and Rubash	Group I	Extraarticular, undisplaced*
	Group II	Extraarticular, displaced*
	Group III	Severely displaced (loss of cortical contact) or angulated
Chen et al	Type I	Nondisplaced(Neer I)
	Type II	Displaced or comminuted (Neer I or II)

Table 3. Classification of supracondylar femoral fractures above total knee arthroplasty reprinted from Su ET, De Wal H, Di Cesare P. Periprosthetic Femoral Fractures Above Total Knee Replacements J Am Acad Orthop Surg, 2004; 12:12 – 20. - with permission (personal communication)

For identifying fracture displacement and deciding whether reduction is needed *Rorabeck et al.* [18] created classification that takes into account both the status of the prosthesis (intact or failing) and the displacement of the fracture:

Type I: fracture is undisplaced and the prosthesis is intact; Type II: fracture is displaced and the prosthesis is intact; Type III: fracture is displaced or undisplaced and the prosthesis is loose or failing

Summarizing above mentioned classifications, we strongly support suggested and explained in article by *Su et al.*[4] which is transcripted (Figure 2)

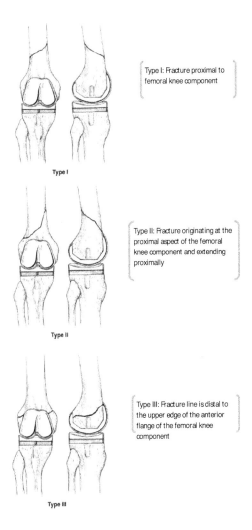

Type I: Fracture proximal to femoral knee component

Type I

Type II: Fracture originating at the proximal aspect of the femoral knee component and extending proximally

Type II

Type III: Fracture line is distal to the upper edge of the anterior flange of the femoral knee component

Type III

Figure 2. Reprinted from Su ET, De Wal H, Di Cesare P. Periprosthetic Femoral Fractures Above Total Knee Replacements J Am Acad Orthop Surg, 2004; 12:12 – 20. - with permission (personal communication)

6. Treatment options

The treatment of supracondylar fractures of the femur following total knee replacement has been a challenge for the orthopaedic surgeon, regardless the fracture and type of fixation [19, 20, 21, 22]. The major goal of treatment should be the restoration of the prefracture functional status of the patient which is characterized by: fracture union, preservation of prosthetic components without loosening, infection and other complications, maintenance of appropriate prosthetic alignment, restoration of joint range of motion. The need to meet all of these objectives makes these fractures difficult to treat: if even single goal is not achieved, the results of treatment will be suboptimal and may lead to failure of the prosthesis. There are two main treatment options: closed (without implant revision) or open (with implant revision), each with various modalities (Tables 4,5) [23, 24, 25, 26].

Skeletal traction
Application of a cast
Pins and plaster
Cast bracing

Table 4. Options for closed treatment of periprosthetic supracondylar femoral fractures

Use of condylar plate
Intramedullary fixation (flexible or rigid, interlocking)
Revision total knee arthroplasty
External fixation
Cerclage wiring with strut allograft fixation
Arthrodesis

Table 5. Options for open treatment of periprosthetic supracondylar femoral fractures

While fracture configuration influences the choice of open versus closed treatment method, fracture displacement, the degree of osteopenia, and the type and technical specifications of the prosthetic components are most valuable determinants of the operative fracture management. Treatment results are closely associated with postfracture alignment and stability [27]. Fracture displacement, intercondylar extension and comminution are negative prognostic factors. High malunion rates are common in association with varus, flexion and internal rotation deformities typically seen as a result of forces exerted by the adductor and gastrocnemius muscle group. Varus femoral malunion is associated with a risk of premature failure of the total knee arthroplasty. The choice of operative treatment method should be based on the patient's health, fracture configuration and displacement, presence of comminution, severity of osteopenia and status of the prosthetic components (loose, unstable or malaligned)[28, 29].

7. Nonoperative treatment

The advantages of nonoperative treatment are: noninvasiveness and negligible infection rate. Since fracture union is likely in nondisplaced fractures, nonoperative treatment is uniformly recommended as the initial management in these cases. Disadvantages include: a relatively high malunion rate and functional loss, particularly in patients with displaced fracture through osteopenic bone in whom maintance of reduction is difficult. Nonoperative treatment is best reserved for nondisplaced fractures that do not demonstrate intercondylar extension. Non-surgical management does eliminate surgical risks such as bleeding, infection, loss of fixation and anesthetic complications. On the other hands, prolonged recumbency in elderly patients carries the significant risk of decubitus ulcers, pneumonia, pulmonary embolia, deep venous thrombosis and diffuse muscle atrophy [30].

8. Operative treatment

Management of periprosthetic fractures of the femur above total knee arthroplasty depends on displacement at the fracture site, bone quality, size of distal fragment and condition of implants (Table 6) [31, 32, 33, 34].

Fracture type	Description of fracture	Treatment recommendation
I	Undisplaced fracture and well fixed prosthesis	Bracing, nonweightbearing
II	Displaced fracture and well fixed prosthesis Good quality bone	Internal fixation using conventional plate, intramedullary nail or locking plate
	Poor quality bone with osteopenia and comminution	Intramedullary nail or locking plate
	Decent size distal fragment Extremely distal fracture	Locking plate or buttress plate with strut allograft
III	Displaced fracture, loose prosthesis No metahyseal bone loss	Revision knee arthroplasty using a long stemmed femoral implant
	Metaphyseal bone loss or nonunion following previous surgery	Structural allograft prosthesis composite or distal femoral replacement prosthesis

Table 6. Operative guidelines for the treatment of periprosthetic supracondylar fractures above total knee arthroplasty

Open reduction and fixation with a *condylar plate* provides the potential advantages of anatomical reconstruction, rigid fixation and an early range of motion exercise. Maintenance of reduction can be a problem, particularly when a patient has a comminuted fracture through osteopenic bone, and malunion is commonly observed. Use of condylar plate is best reserved for less comminuted, displaced fractures with satisfactory bone stock. Using the *buttress condylar plate* include the ability to place the multiple screws distally in many directions and excellent visualization of the fracture to obtain an anatomic reduction. Disadvantages include extensive soft tissue stripping and less rigid fixation than with a nail or fixed angle condylar plate.

Use of *flexible intramedullary rods* is an efficient and less invasive treatment option, although shortening and rotational malunion occasionally occur as a result of the reduced axial and rotational stability. This technique should be considered for mildly displaced fractures patients with unstable general condition. It is minimally invasive procedure with limited morbidity.

New *locking plates* offer advantages over conventional plates for the treatment of periprosthetic fracture associated with total knee arthroplasty. These devices provide stable fixation in osteopenic bone, they are adaptable to different types of fracture and prosthesis and can be inserted using a minimally invasive approach. These plates are particularly useful in presence of an implant in proximal femur as it allows unicortical screw fixation if there is overlapping the distal part of the proximal implant, thus avoiding a stress riser between the two implants.

Rigid supracondylar interlocking rod fixation offers the advantage of being minimally invasive while providing good axial, angular and rotational stability. It can be performed with use of minimal patellar tendon splitting approach with percutaneous placement of interlocking screws in cases with lesser comminution with maintenance of the fracture hematoma and osseous blood supply. Contraindications include loose total knee components, severe comminution, extremely distal fracture and a presence of long total hip intramedullary stem,. This technique has several advantages over traditional open reduction with plate fixation: intramedullary implants are biomechanically superior to subperiostally placed fixation devices, who have significantly larger bending moments; there is no need for periosteal stripping, which can compromise blood supply to the fracture site and increase the risk of nonunion; plate fixation can be technically demanding and often requires the use of supplemental bone grafting.

Revision total knee arthroplasty provides the advantage of stable fixation with a dyaphisis engaging intramedullary femoral stem, allowing early range of motion and weight bearing. This technique is selected for extremely distal or comminuted fractures when stable fixation is difficult to secure with other methods, or for any fracture associated with loose, unstable, or substantially malaligned total knee components. Revision total knee arthroplasty is frequently required in cases where other methods, nonoperative or operative, have failed.

The most difficult cases involve a loose prosthesis coupled with deficient metaphyseal bone stock, rendering a basic revision procedure impossible. Such cases require excision of distal fracture fragment and replacement with either a *distal femoral replacement prosthesis* or a *structural allograft*. These treatment methods may also be required for nonunion resulting from failed osteosynthesis. Distal femoral replacement implants should be considered as a limb salvage option when other surgical options are not feasible. The use of stemmed constrained revision component with structural distal femoral allograft composite has been described as the effective means of providing both implant and fracture stability.

Periprosthetic fractures have a higher rate of nonunion than other supracondylar femoral fractures in the elderly. This has been attributed to alterations in vascularity at the fracture site due to primary surgery, the presence of metal implant and intramedullary polymethyl methacrylate (PMMA), or long term oral corticosteroid administration.

The goals of treatment, whether surgical or nonsurgical, are fracture healing, restoration and maintenance of knee range of motion, and pain free ambulation. A good result is a minimum of 90 degrees of knee motion, with femoral shortening less then 2 cm, varus/valgus malalignment less than 5 degrees, and flexion/extension malalignment less than 10 degrees. Fulfillment of these criteria enables satisfactory knee function, which is of paramout importance to the patient.

9. Complications

Major early complications include nonunion and malunion, which often lead to prosthetic loosening, pain and revision. The treatment of delayed unions with bone grafting is possible and is advocated if appropriate limb alignment and fracture fixation are maintained. In cases of deformity, early signs of prosthetic failure or inability to secure rigid fixation, revision may be the most appropriate. The most devastating complication of operative care of these fractures is infection. Incidence of periprosthetic fracture following total knee arthroplasty is gradually increasing, and management of these fractures can be challenging with complications that severely influence both the patient and surgeon. Furthermore, treatment complication rate range from 20 to 75 percent according to literature data [35]: in a review of 415 cases, there were reported a nonunion rate of 9%, fixation failure in 4%, an infection rate of 3% and revision surgery rate of 13%. Following case will demonstrate some of these problems in treating supracondylar periprosthetic femoral fractures.

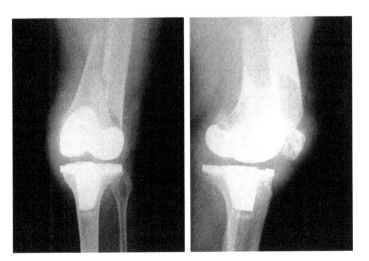

Figure 3. Anteroposterior and lateral view of type II supracondylar femoral fracture

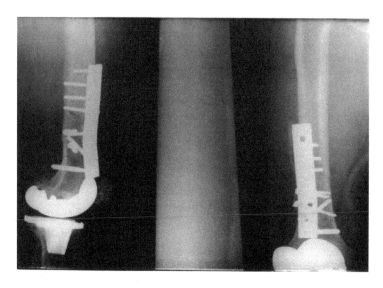

Figure 4. Operative treatment with DCP (anatomic reduction with rigid fixation)

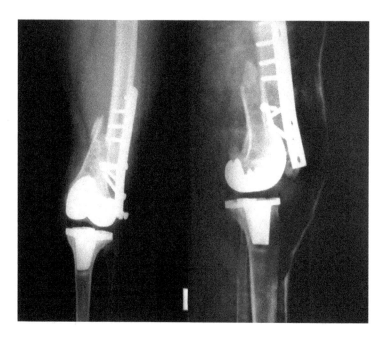

Figure 5. Loss of reduction and fixation two months following surgery

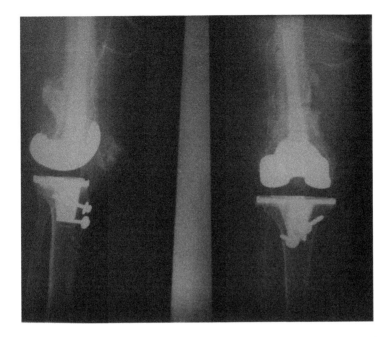

Figure 6. Revision total knee arthroplasty for loose femoral component and fracture treatment

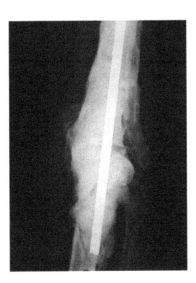

Figure 7. Devastating complication, infection, and limb salvage procedure with antibiotic cement spacer

10. Aftertreatment, rehabilitation

Rehabilitation process is generally guided by the characteristics of the fracture and chosen treatmen methods. As previously said, non-operative treatment is reserved for nondisplaced supracondylar fractures with stable implant and includes longer rehabilitation period to achieve patient's preambulatory status, if it is possible at all. Since surgery and more stable implants including intramedullary nails and angular locking plates allow for faster aftertreatment program, rehabilitation protocol is similar to post fracture treatment in cases without knee arthroplasty. Main goals are fracture healing, implant stability and prefracture functional status.

11. Prevention

Since supracondylar femoral fractures above total knee arthroplasty are mostly seen in osteoporotic patients, prevention of osteopenia and osteoporosis including treatment with bisphosphonate and regular exercise will be good for the well-being of the patient and implant. Surgical factors, such as anterior femoral notching, bone cement hypovascularisation and termal necrosis, and uncontrolled soft tissue manipulation should be kept in mind on regular basis in order to minimize surgeon's impact on development of potential complications including supracondylar fracture.

12. Conclusion

Periprosthetic femoral fractures above total knee prosthesis are increasing complication with constantly growing incidence since the number of total knee replacements and population agings are convergating factors. Risk factors analysis and prevention should be in surgeon and patient focus on this topic. Treatment options include first step to establish whether the implant is loose and, if so even if the fracture is well aligned and heals, treatment that does not include revision will lead to poor result. Prefracture misalignment, osteolysis and polyethylene wear are important factors in the decision making process. The second step in the treatment is to identify fracture displacement and to decide whether reduction is needed. The most appropriate criteria of acceptable fracture alignment are for supracondylar fractures without knee prosthesis: less than 5 mm of translation; less than 5 to10 degrees of angulation; less than 10 mm of shortening and less than 10 degrees of rotational displacement. Any alteration in limb axis resulting from fracture can result in altered loading of the prosthesis, which may in turn lead to enhanced wear and/or accelerated implant loosening. The goals of treatment, whether surgical or nonsurgical, are fracture healing, restoration and maintenance of knee range of motion, and pain free ambulation. A good result is a minimum of 90 degrees of knee motion, with femoral shortening less then 2 cm, varus/valgus malalignment less than 5 degrees, and flexion/extension malalignment less than 10 degrees. Fulfillment of these criteria enables satisfactory knee function, which is of paramout importance to the patient.

Acknowledgements

This work is supported by grant number III 41004, Ministry of Education and Science Republic of Serbia.

Author details

Vladan Stevanović[1*], Zoran Vukašinović[1,2], Zoran Baščarević[1,2], Branislav Starčević[2,3], Dragana Matanović[2,4] and Duško Spasovski[1,2]

*Address all correspondence to: vladanstevanovi90@gmail.com

1 Institute for Orthopaedic Surgery „Banjica", Belgrade, Serbia

2 Faculty of Medicine, University of Belgrade, Belgrade, Serbia

3 Clinic for Orthopaedic Surgery and Traumatology, Clinical Center of Serbia, Belgrade, Serbia

4 Clinic for Physical Therapy and Rehabilitation, Clinical Center of Serbia, Belgrade, Serbia

References

[1] Neer, C. S I. I, Grantham, S. A, & Shelton, M. L. Supracondylar fracture of the adult femur: A study of one hundred and ten cases. J Bone Joint Surge Am (1967). , 49, 591-613.

[2] Culp, R. W, Schmidt, R. G, Hanks, G, & Mak, A. Esterhai JL Jr, Heppenstall RB. Supracondylar fracture of the femur following prosthetic knee arthroplasty. Clin Orthop (1987). , 222, 212-22.

[3] Sisto, D. J, Lachiewicz, P. F, & Insall, J. N. Treatment of supracondylar fractures following prosthetic arthroplasty of the knee. Clin Orthop (1985). , 196, 265-72.

[4] Su, E. T, & De Wal, H. Di Cesare P. Periprosthetic Femoral Fractures Above Total Knee Replacements. J Am Acad Orthop Surg (2004). , 12, 12-20.

[5] Hirsch, D. M, Bhalla, S, & Roffman, M. Supracondylar fracture of the femur following total knee replacement. Report of four cases. J Bone Joint Surg Am (1981). , 63, 162-3.

[6] Lesh, M. L, Schneider, D. J, Deol, G, Davis, B, Jacobs, C. R, & Pellegrini, V. D. The consequences of anterior femoral notching in total knee arthroplasty: a biomechanical study. J Bone Joint Surg Am (2000). , 82, 1096-101.

[7] Dennis, D. A. Periprosthetic fractures following total knee arthroplasty: the good, bad and ugly. Orthopedics (1998). , 21, 1048-50.

[8] Scott, R. D. Anterior femoral notching and ipsilateral supracondylar femur fracture in total knee arthroplasty. J Arthroplasty (1988).

[9] Shawen, S. B. Belmont PJ Jr, Klemme WR, Topoleski LDT, Xenos JS, Orchowski JR. Osteoporosis and anterior femoral notching in periprosthetic supracondylar fractures. A biomechanical study. J Bone Joint Surg Am (2003). , 85, 115-21.

[10] Dennis, A. D. Periprosthetic fractures following total knee arthroplasty. J Bone Joint Surg Am (2001). , 83, 120-4.

[11] Ritter, M. A, Faris, P. M, & Keating, E. M. Anterior femoral notching and ipsilateral supracondylar femur fracture in total knee arthroplasty. J Arthroplasty (1988). , 3, 185-7.

[12] Henry, S. L. Booth RE Jr. Management of supracondylar fractures above total knee prosthesis. Tech Orthop (1995). , 9, 243-52.

[13] Merkel, K. D. Johnson EW Jr. Supracondylar fracture of the femur after total knee arthroplasty. J Bone Joint Surg Am (1986). , 68, 29-43.

[14] Aaron, R. K, & Scott, R. Supracondylar fracture of the femur after total knee arthroplasty. Clin Orthop (1987). , 219, 136-9.

[15] Dennis, D. A. Periprosthetis fractures following total knee arthroplasty. Tech Orthop (1999). , 14, 138-43.

[16] DiGioia AM 3d, Rubash HE. Periprosthetic fractures of the femur after total knee arthroplasty. A literature review and treatment algorithm. Clin Orthop (1991). , 271, 135-42.

[17] Rorabeck, C. H, Angliss, R. D, & Lewis, P. L. Fractures of the femur, tibia and patella after total knee arthroplasty: decision making and principles of management. Instr Course Lect (1998). , 47, 449-60.

[18] Rorabeck, C. H, & Taylor, J. W. Classification of periprosthetic fractures complicating total knee arthroplasty. Orthop Clin North Am (1999). , 30, 209-14.

[19] Shatzker, J, & Lambert, D. C. Supracondylar fractures of the femur. Clin Orthop (1979). , 138, 77-83.

[20] Insall, J. M. Fractures in the distal femur. In: Insall JM, editor. Surgery of the knee. New York: Churchill Livingstone, (1984). , 413-48.

[21] Hohl, M. Fractures about the knee. In: Rockwood CA, Green DP, editors. Fractures in adults.. Philadelphia: JB Lippincott,(1984). , 1478-9.

[22] Rorabeck, C. H, & Taylor, J. W. Periprosthetic fractures of the femur complicating total knee arthroplasty. Orthop Clin North Am (1999). , 30, 265-77.

[23] Harloww, M. L, & Hofmann, A. A. Periprosthetic fractures. In: Scot WN, editor. The knee. St Louis: CV Mosby, (1994). , 1405-17.

[24] Sochart, D. H, & Hardinge, K. Nonsurgical management of supracondylar fracture above total knee arthroplasty. Still the nineties option. J Arthroplasty (1997). , 12, 830-4.

[25] Ayers, D. C. Supracondylar fracture of the distal femur proximal to a total knee replacement. Instr Course Lect (1997). , 46, 197-203.

[26] Chmell, M. J, Moran, M. C, & Scott, R. D. Periarticular fractures after total knee arthroplasty: principles of management. J Am Acad Orthop Surg (1996). , 4, 109-16.

[27] Figgie, M. P, & Goldberg, V. M. Figgie HE III. The results of treatment of supracondylar fracture above total knee arthroplasty. J Arthroplasty (1990). , 5, 267-76.

[28] Kang Il KimEgol KA, Hozack WJ, Parvizi J. Periprosthetic fractures after total knee arthroplasties. Clin Orthop (2006). , 446, 167-75.

[29] Chen, F, Mont, M. A, & Bachner, R. S. Management of ipsilateral supracondylar femuir fractures following total knee arthroplasty. J Arthroplasty (1994). , 9, 521-6.

[30] Sochart, D. H, & Hardinge, K. Nonsurgical management of supracondylar fracture above total knee arthroplasty. Still the nineties option. J Arthroplasty (1997). , 12, 830-4.

[31] Engh, G. A, & Ammeen, D. J. Periprosthetic fractures adjacent to total knee implants. Treatment and clinical results. J Bone Joint Surg Am (1997). , 79, 1100-13.

[32] Cusick, R. P, Lucas, G. L, Mcqueen, D. A, & Graber, C. D. Construct stiffness of different fixation methods for supracondylar femoral fractures above total knee prosthesis. Am J Orthop (2000). , 29, 695-9.

[33] Lewis, P. L, & Rorabeck, C. H. Periprosthetic fractures. In: Engh GA, Rorabeck CH, editors. Revision total knee arthroplasty. Baltimore MD: Williams & Willkins; (1997). , 275-295.

[34] Kolb, K, Grützner, P. A, Marx, F, & Kolb, W. Fixation of Periprosthetic Supracondylar Femur Fractures Above Total Knee Arthroplasty- The Indirect Reduction Technique with the Condylar Blade Plate and the Minimally Invasive Technique with the LISS. In: Fokter S, editor. Recent Advances in Hip and Knee Arthroplasty. Rijeka: InTech, (2012). , 315-42.

[35] Herrera, D. A, Kregor, P. J, Cole, P. A, Levy, B. A, Jonssos, A, & Zlowodzki, M. Treatment of acute distal femur fractures above a total knee arthroplasty: systematic revew of 415 cases (1981-2006). Acta Orthop (2008). , 79, 22-7.

Chapter 4

Extensor Mechanism Complications After Patellar Resurfacing in Knee Replacement – Can They Justify Non-Patellar Resurfacing?

Antonio Silvestre, Raúl Lopez, Fernando Almeida,
Pablo Renovell, Francisco Argüelles and
Oscar Vaamonde

Additional information is available at the end of the chapter

1. Introduction

Patellar resurfacing is still nowadays a controversial matter in articles, cross fires and meetings. We know that this is not a new subject as the issue of whether or not to resurface the patella when performing a TKA has been a debatable topic for more than two decades [1]. We can find three philosophies around what to do with the patella in TKA and there is still no best conclusion about benefits from one or another procedure.

Many randomised trials provide inconclusive evidence in relation to resurface or not the patella after TKA and these trials fail mainly because short sample sizes. Some meta-analysis have been reported last years in order to clarify this issue and though no great differences have been found between both procedures, patellar resurfacing shows better functional results and less anterior knee pain [2-4]. Nevertheless, what is cleared stated in literature is that treatment of the patellofemoral joint in knee replacement and its ultimate results are multifactorial.

Surgeons around the world can be classified into three groups according to their preference in the topic of resurfacing or not the patella: universal resurfacers, non-resurfacers and selective resurfacers. One of the reasons that non-resurfacers use as justification for their performance is that patellar resurfacing implies complications related to extensor mechanism of the knee. Moreover complications related to extensor mechanism are a common basis for

TKA revisions and these problems have less favourable outcome than patients who undergo revision for other reasons.

The use of computer-aid navigation systems in knee replacement have allowed to accurate some of the mistakes in coronal, sagittal and axial alignment of femoral and tibial implant that are related to patellar maltracking. In the near future it should be possible to navigate the patellofemoral joint, so problems linked to this compartment will diminish. Until now, there is a report of a surgical navigation system that let to assess intraoperatively patellar tracking, one of the main reasons of TKAs' failure, with the aid of a computer. The system is quite complex and it is not available for all the knee prosthesis designs. However, the method could be a valuable support to analyze patellar tracking at the time of the surgery and a real help to decide whether or not patellar replacement [5].

In this study we have reviewed our extensor mechanism complications relate to knee replacement for the last 6 years in order to analyze if they have a high rate that could justify non-patellar resurfacing. We believe that a careful and meticulous technique during patellar resurfacing can avoid most of the problems found after knee replacement. It is not reasonable that in these days in which many surgeons are worried about accurate alignment of knee components and most of them use computer-aid navigation systems to be more precise in prosthesis placement we are not as careful as in other steps of the procedure when resurfacing the patella.

2. Material and method

We have retrospectively revised all the TKA's performed in our Institution from January 2005 until December 2011. For this period of time, the two fellowship-trained surgeons (AS and FA) performed 860 TKA using a standard technique for knee replacement and similar rehabilitation protocol. Postero-stabilized cemented total knee arthroplasties were used in all cases (Performance® Biomet Warsaw, IN and Vanguard® Biomet Warsaw, IN). Patella was resurfaced in all cases according to the philosophy of our Department. Demographic data are shown in table I.

A single dose of intravenous antibiotic (cefazolin 2 gr or vancomycin 1gr in allergic patients according to the protocol of our Hospital Infection Control Committee) was given ½ hour before incision. After general o regional anaesthesia depending on patient and physician's preference, tourniquet was routinely applied as proximal as possible in the thigh. Longitudinal incision along the knee and medial para-patellar arthrotomy were performed to gain access to the joint. Surgery was performed according to the standard procedure and femur and tibial implants were cemented to the bone. Careful alignment of both components was checked before implantation. Posterior-condyle plus 3° of external rotation and trans-epicondylar axis were used without distinction to get an adequate femoral rotation. On the other hand tibial component was aligned to the medial third of the tibial tubercle. We don't usually evert the patella during this time of the procedure. Once femoral and tibial trials were in place, we arrange for the patellar resurfacing step.

Sex	Female: 536/ Male: 324
Side	Right: 492/ Left: 368
Age (years)	73.15±6.06
BMI (kg/m²)	27.76±3.12
Previous surgery (%)	38.3%
Radiological valgus (%)	9.7%
Pre-operative diagnoses	
Osteoarthritis	593
Osteonecrosis medial condyle	137
Metabolic arthritis	78
RA	35
Fracture sequela	17

Table 1. Demographic data and preoperative parameters

In our experience it is crucial to be as thorough as possible in patellar resurfacing step to achieve good results and avoid extensor mechanism complications. Most of these problems should be avoid with a more methodical procedure. We employ the instruments provide by the manufacturer to afford patellar resurfacing though we accept they are not always useful. However, more precise instruments in recent systems allow more accuracy placing the patella. The Vanguard System Knee® provides specifically devices (cutting guide) to improve the results. It offers a calliper or vernier to estimate patella thickness before and after the cut, a guide with a magnetize gauge to determine the deep of the cut after guide positioning and it is possible to choose single or three-peg configuration at the time of the surgery. Devices availability in theatre make the surgeons more self-assured when dealing with patello-femoral joint. Albeit these devices can't be employed in 100% of cases as patellar morphology, size or wear difficult its use. The fact that surgical instrumental can't be employed, doesn't mean patellar resurfacing is a trivial step in knee surgery.

For this series we have used all-polyethylene patellar component design with single or three-peg configuration. The prostheses employed in our cases just provide onlay patellar implants. We usually make peripheral electrocautery around the patella and remove soft-tissue synovium in the upper part of the patella to avoid patellar clunk syndrome as we perform posterior stabilized designs.

Patients received intravenous antibiotics (cefazolin 1g/8h) for 48 h after surgery according to the protocol of our Institution. Post-operative bandage was removed at the second day after surgery to check incision and vascular condition of the leg. Output drainage was removed 36-48 h after surgery. They started physiotherapy of the operated knee the second day after surgery when drains were removed if proper laboratory values were obtained. Full weight bearing on the operated limb was allowed immediately except in those cases the surgeon contraindicated the pre-established protocol because of surgical difficulties. Physiothera-

Extensor Mechanism Complications After Patellar Resurfacing in Knee Replacement – Can They Justify Non-Patellar Resurfacing?

75

pists instructed the patients to walk either with walker or crutches depending on their ability. They go up stairs with the help of the banister the fourth-fifth day after surgery before leaving the Hospital.

Prophylactic low molecular weight heparin (enoxaparin) was used for the next 28 days after surgery. Patients stay at our Institution depends on his/her ability to keep up with daily activities (range 4-8 days), obviously after their haematological values were as best as possible.

Outpatient follow-up was done at 6, 12 weeks and the annually for clinical and radiological evaluation of the operated knee. We assessed clinical evaluation including gait, need for assistance devices, ROM, joint stability, knee score (KSS) and visual analog scale (VAS). Routine A-P and lateral views were done to evaluate mechanical axis and proper alignment of the implant. In those cases with extensor mechanism complications axial views and other techniques such as US, CT or MR were used to analyze the problem.

Intra-operative and post-operative complications were captured and collected for descriptive study. Arthroscopic technique was indicated in case internal injuries of the knee (patellar clunk syndrome); on the other hand open surgery was used for management of instabilities, tendon ruptures, patellar fracture…

3. Results

There were 860 primary total knee arthroplasties performed with the use of the "Performance System" (Biomet®, Warsaw, IN) and the "Vanguard System" (Biomet®, Warsaw, IN) in this series, done through a longitudinal incision with medial para-patellar arthrotomy. Underlying diagnosis was osteoarthritis and osteonecrosis of the medial condyle in more than 80% of cases. Mean follow-up was 48 months (ranging from 6 to 78 months).

Thirteen patients (1.51%) showed wound infection and developed an acute infection and eleven cases (1.27%) suffered haematogenous infection more than a year after surgery so these patients were excluded from this series as they required revision surgery (836 patients were included in this series). Co-morbidities in these patients were diabetes mellitus, rheumatoid arthritis and obesity. During follow-up elevated ESR (>20) and CRP (>5) values and clinical signs of infection were detected. Aspiration culture was positive 19 cases (79.16%) and the most frequent microorganisms identified were staphylococcus spp, meticillin-resistant staphylococcus aureus, streptococcus spp and pseudomona aeuruginosa.

In our series required time to walk by a walker or two crutches was 2.25±1.45 days and patients were able to go up and down stairs with the help of the banister at 5.03±2.67 days (range 4-15 days). More than sixty percent of patients were capable to walk without the help of any assistive aids at four weeks postoperatively. However, we advise the use of at least one cane for the first six weeks after the operation, to avoid stumbling as many patients in this series are elderly. Clinical results are shown in table II.

Knee Society Score improved from 53.48±6.21 (range 39-67) to 92.037± 7.23 (range 85-94) a year after surgery. Visual analog pain score after surgery improved to 1.891±0.31 in more than 90% of cases three months after surgical procedure. This can be judge as a satisfactory score as painful knee arthroplasty is a non-desired state after joint reconstruction.

		Preoperative	6 weeks	12 weeks	1 year
Pain (VAS)	<2 (%)	2.39	83.61	92.19	94.49
	2 to <5 (%)	35.52	13.63	5.75	3.96
	5 to <8 (%)	45.09	2.51	1.91	1.31
	>8%	17	0.24	0.24	0.24
KSS (knee score)		53.48±6.21	79.437±8.32	89.065±5.87	92.037±7.23
Average ROM		-5 /85°	0 /95°	0 / 115°	0 / 115°
Walking capability	>2 h (%)	1.91	50.35	60.04	61.96
	>1 h (%)	22	27.63	29.06	29.06
	>30' (%)	75	31.31	10.43	8.51
	Not walk (%)	1.09	0.71	0.47	0.47
Walking support	No support (%)	57.05	62.53	86.12	90.55
	1 cane or crutch (%)	42	35.81	12.58	8.27
	2 crutches (%)	0.95	0.95	0.83	0.71
Stairs	Normal (%)	63.03	77.25	85.16	85.52
	Banister (%)	35.88	21.54	14.37	14.01

Table 2. Clinical results

Mechanical axis (180°±3°) was restored in 95.04% of cases. Alignments of the femoral and tibial implants in frontal and coronal axes were measured without significant deviation from standard values.

Main extensor mechanism complications are shown in table III. The most frequent complications were instability of the extensor mechanism and patellar fractures. However, most of the fractures were related to a traumatic event as patients in this series were old people, so this complication cannot be only linked to surgical aggression. Patellar tendon rupture was mostly related to knees with previous surgery as valgus osteotomy.

Instability of the extensor mechanism (patellar dislocation or subluxation)	1.79% (15 cases)
Patellar fracture	1.43% (12 cases)
Patellar tendon rupture	0.47% (4 cases)
Patella loosening	0.95% (8 cases)
Clunk syndrome	0.71 (6 cases)

Table 3. Extensor mechanism complications

4. Discussion

For many years dealing with the patella in total knee arthroplasties has been a controversial topic. Most of the non-resurfacers surgeons justify their choice based in the frequent complications related to surgery around the patella. It is true that surgical gestures used during patellar resurfacing can affect the patello-femoral tracking, weak patellar bone or alter vascularisation around the patella. Besides it has been remarked by many authors that some knee replacements failures are related to disorders in the mechanics of the patellofemoral joint.

Soft-tissue imbalance is shown as the responsible of patellar instability, the most frequent extensor mechanism complication with an incidence as high as 29% in some series after TKAs [6]. Muscle atrophy, weakness, more proximal attachment of the VMO after closure of the arthrotomy and predominance of the VL are considered the main causes of patellofemoral dysfunction [6]. However, forces from the different bellies of the quadriceps can modify patellofemoral function [7].

Aside from anatomical aspects of the quadriceps that are non surgical-dependant, some technical aspects on the patellar side should be observed during this step of the surgery. It is of main importance to restore patellar thickness to prevent from high mechanical pressures and increase de risk of patellar fracture [8]. It is recommended to maintain between 13 and 15 mm of patellar bone remained to adapt the all-polyethylene insert which has 8-10 mm thickness. Surgical technique is of crucial importance in patellar alignment. An increase combined thickness of the implant and patellar bone leads to higher forces on patellar side and close follow-up of these patients should be done. Postoperative lateral tilt increased when thickness after patella resurfacing was augment in 1 mm from the preoperative patella [9]. This lateral tilt is usually treated by lateral release that improves patellar alignment, but lateral release is related to complications as patellar fracture, vascular problems and postoperative pain [10].

Patellar fracture is not an exclusive complication of resurfaced patella and can be sustained in non-resurfaced cases but in rates as low as 0.05%. They are usually related to rheumatoid arthritis or advanced degenerative osteoarthritis [11]. Only in cases of a thin patella or sclerotic bone we advise not to resurface the patella.

Another important fact in this patellar reconstruction is the direction of the osteotomy. Changes in resection angle influence patellar tracking and favour lateral tilt that could require a subsequent lateral release. The goal is to get a flat bone cut with a symmetrical resection. This step could be done freehand, but we employ the cutting guide provides by the manufacturer to improve our results. Once the cut has been done, medial placement of the polyethylene offers better patellar tracking than if it is placed laterally. It is advisable to assess patellar tracking with the "no-thumb" rule placing the knee through full ROM. If the patella tracks laterally, lateral release should be taken into account trying to preserve superior lateral genicular vessels in order to avoid osteonecrosis, patellar fracture or post-operative pain [8, 10].

The fixation of the implant could be done with single or three pegs system depending on surgeon's preference. Today loosening of the patella is a rare complication. As we have said our knee models have only available "onlay" patellar prosthesis, though some authors recommend "inlay" inserts which make them more confident, but no significant differences are observed between the two models [12]. It is said that "inlay" implants allow increase the interface bone-cement, preserve more bone stock and are easy to use [13], but survivorship and clinical and radiological results are similar to the "onlay" designs [14]. In our series we have employed all-polyethylene patella without important complications and good functional outcomes.

Patellar instability, which may happen after TKA with or without patellar resurfacing, is a major cause of functional restraint that requires revision surgery. The incidence of symptomatic instability leading to revision is around 0.8%, lower than instability of the extensor mechanism in our series, but we want to remark that most of our cases were classified as subluxations (8 cases out of 15), not frank dislocations so revision rate was similar. Conservative methods as quadriceps exercises, braces or avoiding activities that aggravate instability were applied in subluxations and with time scarring of the retinacular tissues lead to resolutions of the symptoms. However in cases of frank dislocation revision surgery was mandatory. In these cases careful analysis of prosthesis sources of instability were cautious checked to avoid failed surgery. If problem was related to soft tissues, realignment of the extensor mechanism should be considered (lateral release plus proximal or distal realignment) [15].

We must remember that other issues as design and placement of the implants may predispose to extensor mechanism complications. Design of the femoral sulcus generated years ago high incidence of patellofemoral complications and led to debate if patella should be resurface and how to do this replacement [16]. Modern knee prostheses have got more anatomic designs, but even now there is no consensus about the size, shape and position of the femoral trochlea in relation to femorotibial compartment [17]. Furthermore it is important to restore sulcus position (0.7 mm lateral to the midline of the distal femoral cut) during surgery as best as possible [18].

As well as properties of the femoral and patellar designs, surgical details of the technique are also valuables. Restoration of the mechanical axis is of great importance in knee surgery, as it is selecting the appropriate size of the femur to avoid overstuffing of the anterior compartment [19] and placing the femoral implant lateralized. Femorotibial alignment influen-ces patellar tracking in native knees as does after knee replacement. Navigation systems that allow surgeons to be more precise in coronal and sagittal planes alignment avoid problems in patellofemoral joints [10].

In our opinion getting the proper rotation for the femoral and tibial components is the main goal to avoid complications of the extensor mechanism [19, 20]. There are four ways for de-termining the rotational alignment of the femur, however we have only used in this series the trans-epicondylar axis and 3° of external rotation based on the posterior condyles. Rota-tional alignment of the tibia is as important as femoral placement, so neutral or external ro-tation of the tibial component in relation to the tibia decreases the Q angle and helps patellar tracking [20, 21]. Usually more attention is paid to rotational position of the femoral compo-nent than to the tibial baseplate and the goal to get proper coverage and good cortical sup-port for the tibial implant could led to a wrong rotational tibial alignment. External rotation of the tibial component moves the tibial tubercle internally so less patellofemoral complica-tions are detected in this situation [22]. Precise rotational tibial alignment can be obtained from a line perpendicular to the epicondylar axis of the femur [22].

Significance of implant position is crucial in order to avoid extensor mechanism problems, so navigation or personal guides system should offer some advantages at the time of pros-theses placement. However many authors believe that proper accuracy can be obtain with traditional guides. X-ray allow to evaluate alignment of the components in the coronal and sagittal plane as well as patellar tracking in the axial view, but rotational position of the im-plants can't be assess by simple radiographies. In these cases we must employ CT to get a more precise image of the situation of the components that can justify extensor mechanism complications.

It is important to remark the importance of being careful with this resurfacing step as we are with the other ones. It's surprising as some surgeons are extremely cautious with bone cuts, implant alignment and gaps balancing, but not so watchful with patellar re-surfacing. After patella evertion they made a non-controlled cut and leave the PE com-ponent on it, without taking into account cut direction, bone width or thickness and medialization of the PE implant.

Preoperative patellar tracking can be a measurement of great value in order to analyze pa-tellar position after TKA. Lateral displacement of 3 mm is predictive of patellar maltracking when the knee is placed in full ROM after surgery. This is an evidence of the issue that pa-tellar tracking is related to soft-tissue tension [23]. Lateral shift of the patella implies a con-tracture of the lateral tissues and this event can be detected in standard preoperative radiographic images. This can be help to identify patients at a higher likehood of experienc-ing maltracking after TKA [23]. Of course a valgus knee deformity is related to problems with patellar tracking, but a more careful analysis of the preoperative X-ray may help us in patellar replacement decision.

Resurfacing the patella by all-polyethylene implant can be questioned as this surgical ges-ture obviously affects patellar tracking, but on the other hand non-resurfacing the patella suppose a different pattern of contact at the patellofemoral joint. To assess intraoperatively patellar tracking a surgical navigation system with the aid of a computer have been designed but until now it is not routinely used. However, the system could be a valuable support to analyze one of the main reasons of failure in TKAs [5].

Until recent days it couldn't have been established a correlation between anterior knee pain and weight [24]. However there is some evidence of a relationship between knee pain and patella tilt. [25]. So "inlay" implants have been criticized for leaving a portion of the lateral facet uncovered by the implant that could be considered a source of pain as it articulates with the femoral component. This liaison may be linked to increase anterior knee pain or worse Knee Society Score. Though we have checked few problems with "onlay" insert in our series, some authors prefer the inset technique of patella resurfacing which for them is simple and safe [1]. We have no experience with the inset patella design proposed by Freeman in 1989 and improved over the years. It looks as this design would have less patellar tracking problems, would need less lateral releases and show less signs of instability in the axial X-rays. On the other hand the technique is more demanding and sacrifices more bone, but allow us to be more precise in restoring patellar thickness [1].

Many extensor mechanism complications can be evaluated through simple X-ray (patellofemoral instability, patellar fracture, loosening of the patellar insert, complete patellar o quadricipital tendon rupture...). US images and IRM help us in diagnosis of partial ruptures of the extensor mechanism, synovial effusions... and TC is of great aid in analyzing rotational position of the components. But what can we do in front of a painful total knee arthroplasty without positive results in conventional diagnostic techniques. The easiest decision is to resurface the patella in case it wasn't but if it was? Careful analysis of the different diagnostic tools is essential (X-ray, evaluation of patellar tracking, CT imaging to check components rotation...). Recently SPECT/CT imaging looks very helpful in establishing the diagnosis of painful knees after TKA, mainly when we are in front of patellofemoral problems without components malposition or loosening. A significantly higher tracer uptake in the patella is shown with this SPECT/CT technique in patients with painful knee due to patellofemoral problems [26].

Patella resurfacing is related to good clinical results but is also linked to some extensor mechanism complications and a possible need for revision surgery in the future [25]. On the other hand, non-resurfacing could avoid complications of the extensor mechanism but a high rate of anterior knee pain is perceived. This situation drives the surgeon to a predictable reoperation as patients increase their retrieval of pain relief. For this reason we consider the decision to resurface the patella as a subjective question [25]. Current literature on patellar resurfacing after TKA has not shown a clear advantage of patellar resurfacing if we analyzed clinical scores, though for many authors patellar replacement looks a better strategy in order to avoid reoperation and anterior knee pain. As the average reoperation rate for non-resurfaced cases was 7.2% compared to 2.8% for the resurfaced, resurfacing the patella would prevent one revision surgery for every 23 patella resurfaced. Knowing the cost of a revision surgery and taking into account that less than 50% of patients would benefit from a secondary resurfacing, primary replacement of the patella offers economic and clinical advantages [25].

The Swedish Knee Arthroplasty Registry shows statistically significant patient satisfaction in cases of patella resurfacing in 98% of about 27000 knees follow-up at 14 years. The Registry also shows that there is 1.27 risk ratio for unresurfaced patella to be revised. The Australian National Joint Registry reveals the same risk ratio (1.25). We must be careful with these numbers about unresurfaced patella being revised because our first option in front of a patient with anterior knee pain an unresurfaced patella is to resurface it. However, more than 50% of patients are dissatisfied with revision for only patella component [27, 28]. What looks evident from the different meta-analysis is that anterior knee pain is greater after non-resurfacing the patella, as well as patient dissatisfaction and increase revision rate. It looks positive resurfacing the patella at primary surgery based on functional results [27]. Some authors do not agree with this assertion and after an observational study from the Norwegian Arthroplasty Register they conclude that patella resurfacing has no clinical effect on function or anterior knee pain, which is debatable [29]. The Norwegian Register finds a lower risk of revision when the patella is resurfaced after a TKA although differences in rates of revision surgery are not significant. But improvement in new prosthesis designs that have substituted the older ones has been related to an increase in the survivorship of the knee prosthesis in Norway [30].

In a prospective cohort study that compares resurfaced vs. non-resurfaced patella in 65 patients that received bilateral total knee replacement, significant better scores were achieved on the resurfaced side at final follow-up. Anterior knee pain was a complaint in 4 patients on the non-resurfaced side and revision surgery was required in these patients. On the other hand no revision was performed in the resurfaced side. The author concluded that better patellofemoral functional outcomes, less anterior knee pain and lower rates of revision surgery could be obtained after patella resurfacing [31].

Nowadays, it looks as two great groups of surgeons are completely established and divided by a huge lake: the North American resurfacers and the European non-resurfacers, however it is not possible to reach a conclusion about which alternative is better. But we can add another group whose select when to resurface the patella. Which are their criteria? How can they determine which patients would need or not patellar resurfacing? The quality of the cartilage and joint congruence can be parameters that aid in the determination of selective patellar resurfacing [32, 33]. When could we advise not to resurface the patella? Park et al remark that non-resurfaced patella is possible if the patient is a young one, the patella is small and its cartilage is almost normal, the patient has no preoperative anterior pain and bone quality is good [34]. If some surgeon decides not to resurface the patella it looks advisable to remove osteophytes of the patella and carry a marginal electrocauterization. Selective resurfacing of patellar bone with specific criteria and the used a patella-friendly implant can be associated with satisfactory outcomes [34].

Reasons for resurfacing the patella are avoiding anterior knee pain, so reoperation rate can be reduced, improve results in some patients with RA and improve functional outcomes as going up stairs [35].

The great majority of evidences and experiences are in favour of patellar resurfacing, so we also recommend substituting the patella [36]. This surgical detail only add a short time (less than 8 minutes) to the surgery and warrant less complains of anterior knee pain [35].

However patellar resurfacing no longer should be considered a mandatory step in TKAs. We must consider femoral and patellar design before resurfacing patella as several authors have reported nice results with patella non-resurfacing [37]. The importance of the femoral design (patella-friendly component) is of maximum significance as coupling patella design provides better anterior knee pain results and improved knee functions. Routine patellar re-placement in TKA cannot be defended when a coupling femoral component is available [37]. However, proper femoral component design is necessary in order to compare patellar resur-facing and non-resurfacing.

As we can see many features influence patellofemoral function after TKAs but surgical tech-nique is one the primary factors affecting patellar alignment [10], so we can conclude that surgical technique and accurate placement of the implants are of crucial importance in patel-la resurfacing and a careful procedure improves outcomes.

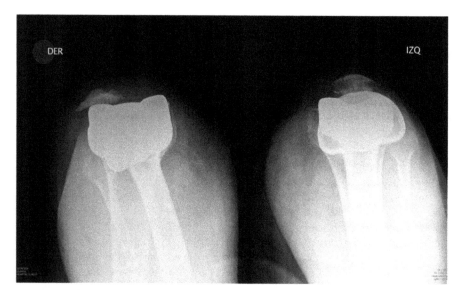

Figure 1. Advanced-age patient suffered subluxation of the extensor mechanism due to a patella infera, after total knee replacement. It was well tolerated; orthopedics measures were employed (a brace and avoiding activities that aggravate instability)

The determination whether to resurface the patella or not is still nowadays controversial [25]. Some trials have concluded there are no advantages in routine patellar resurfacing [38, 39] meanwhile other reports [40] and some meta-analyses [2-4] show less anterior knee pain, better functional outcomes and lower rates of revision after patella resurfacing.

We believe the ultimate result of the patella treatment in total knee replacement is multifactorial and depend on patient factors (illness, previous pain, age, weight, BMI...), surgical technique (features shown before), implant design (trochlear groove, tibial implant, patella size and thickness) and above all a proper placement of the components.

However pain is the main reason why the patients seek for a TKA. They accept undergo this procedure to alleviate pain and to restore as best function as possible. Literature reports better functional results and less pain after patellar resurfacing. It seems not fair to avoid patellar resurfacing for financial criterion or because longer surgical times. If extensor mechanical problems are not as frequent as our series shows and look like these complications could be an acceptable risk, why not to resurface the patella?

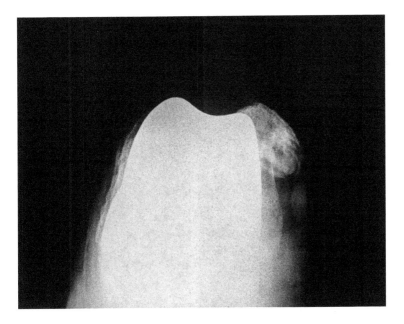

Figure 2. Frank dislocation of the patella who required revision surgery. Internal rotational alignment of the femoral component made us to revise it, getting good functional outcome after surgery.

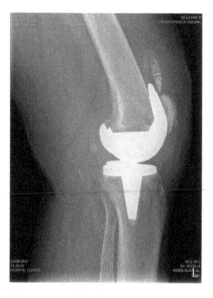

Figure 3. Loosening of the patellar insert that required removing of the polyethylene. As quality of remaining bone wasn't good, no other all-polyethylene implant was placed

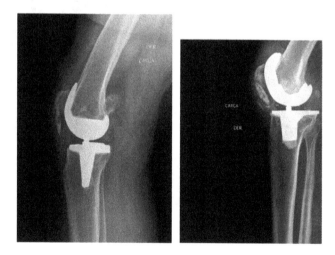

Figure 4. Two examples of fracture of the patella with loosening of the patella. The patients referred a previous trauma in both cases and revision surgery with extensor mechanism reconstruction was done.

Author details

Antonio Silvestre[1,2], Raúl Lopez[1], Fernando Almeida[1], Pablo Renovell[1],
Francisco Argüelles[1] and Oscar Vaamonde[1]

1 Clinic Hospital of Valencia, Spain

2 Orthopedic Department, School of Medicine, University of Valencia, Spain

References

[1] Hurson C, Kashir A, Flavin R, Kelly I. Routine patellar resurfacing using an inset patellar technique. International Orthopaedics, 2010; 34: 955-58

[2] Parvizi J, Rapuri VR, Saleh KJ, Kuskowski MA, Sharkey PF, Mont MA. Failure to resurface the patella during total knee arthroplasty may result in more knee pain and
secondary surgery. Clin Orthop, 2005; 438:191–96

[3] Pakos EE, Ntzani EE, Trikalinos TA. Patellar resurfacing in total knee arthroplasty. A
meta-analysis. J Bone Joint Surg Am, 2005; 87 (7):1438–45

[4] Nizard R S, Biau D, Porcher R, Ravaud P, Bizot P, Hannouche D, Sedel L. A meta-
analysis of patellar replacement in total knee arthroplasty. Clin Orthop 2005; 432:
196-203.

[5] Belvedere C, Catani F, Ensini A, Moctezuma de la Barrera JL, Leardini A. Paellar
Trucking Turing total knee arthroplasty: an in Vitro feasibility stydu. Knee Surg
Sports Traumatol Arthrosc 2007; 15: 985-93

[6] Walligora AC. Johanson NA, Hirsch BE. Clinical Anatomy of the quadriceps femoris
and extensor apparatus of the knee. Clin Orthop. 2009 (467: 3297-306

[7] Amis AA. Current concepts on anatomy and biomechanics of patellar stability.
Sports Med Arthrosc. 2007; 15:48–56

[8] Levai JP. Technical aspects: The patellar side. Knee Surg Sports Traumatol Arthrosc.
2011; 9 (suppl 1): S19-S20

[9] Youm YS, Cho WS, Woo JH, Kim BK. The effect of patellar thickness changes on patellar tilt in total knee arthroplasty. Knee Surg Sports Traumatol Arthrosc. 2010; 18:
923-7

[10] Fukagawa S, Matsuda S, Mizu-uchi H, Miura H, Okazaki K, Iwamoto Y. Cjanges in
patellar alignment alter total knee arthroplasty. Knee Surg Sports Traumtol Arthrosc.
2011; 19: 99-104

[11] Seijas R, Orduña JM, Castro MC, Granados N, baliarda J, Alcantara E. Journal of Or-
thopeadic Surgery 2009; 17(2): 251-4

[12] Freeman MA, Samuelson K-M, Elias S-G, Mariorenzi LJ, Gokcay EI, Tuke M. The patellofemoral joint in total knee prostheses. Design considerations. J Arthroplasty, 1989; 4 [Suppl]:69–74

[13] Rosentein AD, Postak PD, Greenwald AS. Fixation strength comparision of onlay and inset patellar implants. Knee. 2007; 14 (3): 194-7

[14] Erak S, Rajgopal V, Mac Donald SJ, McCalden RW, Burne RB. Ten-year results o fan inset biconvex patella prosthesis in primary knee artrhoplasty. Clin Orthop, 2009; 467: 1781-92

[15] Motsis EK, Paschos N, Pakos EE, Georgoulis AD. Review article: Patellar instability alter total knee arthroplasty. Journal of Orthopaedic Surgesry. 2009; 17 (3):351-7

[16] Kulkarni SK, Freeman MAR, Poal-Manresa JC, Asencio JI, Rodriguez JJ. The patellofemoral Joint in total knee arthroplasty: is the designo f the trochlea the critical factor?. Knee Surg Sports Traumatol Arthrosc. 2001; 9 (Supp 1): S8-S12

[17] Iranpour F, Merican AM, Dandachii W, Amis AA, Cobb JP. The geometry of the trochlear groove. Clin Orthop. 2010; 468: 782-788

[18] Lingaraj K, Bartlett J. The femoral sulcus in total knee artrhoplasty. Knee Surg Sports Traumatol Arthrosc. 2009; 17: 499-502

[19] Gosh KM, Merican AM, Iranpour F, Deehan DJ, Amis AA. The effect of overstuffing the patellofemoral Joint on the extensor retinaculum of the knee. Knee Surg Sports Traumtol Arthrosc, 2009; 17: 1211-16

[20] Anglin C, Brimacombe JM, Hodgson AJ, Masri BA, Greidanus NV, Tonetti J, Wilson DR. Determinants of patellar tracking in total knee arthroplasty. Clin Biomech (Bristol, Avon). 2008; 23:900–910

[21] Luring C, Perlick L, Bathis H, Tingart M, Grifka J The effect of femoral component rotation on patellar tracking in total knee arthroplasty. Orthopedics, 2007; 30:965–967

[22] Rossi R, Bruzzone M, Bonasia DE, Marmottu A, Castoldi F. Evaluation of tibial rotacional alignment in total knee arthroplasty: a cadáver study. Knee Surg Sports Traumatol Arthrosc, 2010; 18: 889-93

[23] Chia SL, Merican AM, Devadasan B, Strachan RK, Amis AA. Radiographic features predicitive of patellar maltracking during total knee arthroplasty. Knee Surg Sports Traumtol Arthrosc 2009; 17: 1217-24

[24] Wood DJ, Smith AJ, Collopy D, White B, Brankov B, Bulsara MK. Patellar resurfacing in total knee arthroplasty: a prospective randomized trial. J Bone Jt Surg Am. 2002; 21 (2): 129-37

[25] Helmy N, Anglin C, Greidanus N, Masri B. To resurface or not resurface the patella in total knee arthroplasty. Clin Orthop, 2008; 466: 2775-83

[26] Hirschmann MT, Konala P, Iranour F, Kerner A, Rasch H, Friederich NF. Clinical value of SPECT/CT for evaluation of patients with painful knees after total knee ar-

throplasty – a new dimension of diagnostics? BMC Musculoskeletal disorders, 2011; 12: 36-46

[27] Clements WJ, Miller S, Whitehouse SL, Graves SE, Ryan P, Crawford RW. Early outcomes of patella resurfacing in total knee arthroplasty. A report from the Australian Orthopaedic Association National Joint Replacement Registry. Acta Orthopaedica 2010; 81 (1): 108-13

[28] Parvizi J, Mortazavi SM, Devulapalli C, Hozack WJ, Sharkey PF, Tithman RH. Secondary resurfacing of the patella after primary total knee arthroplasty does the anterior pain resolve? J Arthroplasty 2012; 27 (1): 21-6

[29] Lygre SHL, Espehaug B, Havelin LI, Vollset SE, Furnes O. Does patella resurfacing really matter? Pain and function in 972 patients alter primary total knee arthroplasty. An observational study from the Norwegian Arthroplasty Register. Acta Ortthopaedica 2010; 81(1): 99-107

[30] Lygre SHL, Espehaug B, Havelin LI, Vollset SE, Furnes O. Failure of total knee arthroplasty with or withpout patella resurfacing. A study from the Norwegian Arthroplasty Register with 0-15 of follow-up. Acta Orthopaedica 2011; 82 (2): 282-92

[31] Patel K, Raut V. Patella in total knee arthroplasty: to resurface or not to – a cohorte study of staged bilateral total knee arthroplasty. International Orthopaedics, 2011; 35: 349-53

[32] Atik OS. Is Soutine patellar resurfacing in total knee arthroplasty necessary?. Eklem Hastalikian ve Cerrahisi, 2010; 21: 61

[33] Sanchez-Marquez JM, Rodriguez-Merchan EC. Implantación del componente rotuliano en la artroplastia total de rodilla: situación actual. Rev esp cir ortop traumatol 2010; 54 (3): 186-92

[34] Se-Jin P, Young-Bok J, Hwa –Jae J, Hun-Kyu S, Ho-Joong J, Jong.Jum L, Ji-Woong Y, Kim E. Long-term results of primary total knee arthroplasty with and without patellar resurfacing. Acta Med Okayama 2010; 64 (5): 331-38

[35] Ghasemzadeh F, Mateescu C. Resurfacing patella in 140 TKA patients. Letter to the editor. IRCMJ, 2010; 12 (1): 76-8

[36] Li S, Chen Y, Su W, Zhao J, He S, Luo X. Systematic review of patellar resurfacing in total knee artrhoplasty. International Orthopaedics, 2011; 35: 305-16

[37] Whitesides LA. Patella resurfacing no longer considered routine in TKA. Orhtopaedics 2006; 29 (9): 833-5

[38] Campbell DG, Duncan WW, Ashworth M, Mintz A, Stirling J, Wakefield L, Stevenson TM. Patellar resurfacing in total knee replacement: a ten-year randomized prospective trial. J Bone Jt Surg Br. 2006; 88 /6): 734-9

[39] Maculé F, castillo F, Llopis-Miró R, Nogales J, Budeus Gonzalez-Solis JM, Lozano LM, Segur JM, Suso S. Sustitución patelar en artroplastia total de rodilla. Estudio prospectivo multicéntrico: resultados preliminares. Avances Traum, 2008; 38 (1): 30-4

[40] Waters TS, Bentley G. Patellar resurfacing in total knee arthroplasty. A prospective randomized study. J Bone Jt Surg Am. 2003 85 (2); 212-7

Chapter 5

Glenoid Loosening in Total Shoulder Arthroplasty

Nahum Rosenberg, Maruan Haddad and
Doron Norman

Additional information is available at the end of the chapter

1. Introduction

Inflammatory or degenerative processes in glenohumeral joint lead to pain and restriction of movements of the shoulder. Prosthetic replacement of the glenohumeral joint has gained in popularity because of its efficacy in relieving pain. The pioneering successful prostheses for total shoulder arthroplasty (TSA) have been based on an unconstrained design, i.e. a metal spherical head component fixed to a metal intramedullary stem articulating with a high-density polyethylene socket. These components are stabilized in the adjacent bone using polymethylmethacrylate (PMMA) bone cement [1]. The most important cause for failure of the cemented prostheses is related to the glenoid component, with a 0.01-6% rate of loosening [2, 3, 4].

The long term survivorship data of the prosthesis developed by C. Neer for the cemented total shoulder arthroplasty (TSA) show 87% fifteen year survivorship rate for Neer I & II cemented shoulder prostheses [5]. This implant has become the gold standard, against which all the successive prosthetic designs are compared.

Further developments of TSA implants have been aimed at enhancing longevity by addressing the following most critical issues: (1) Improving the incorporation of the glenoid component using a more "biological" type of fixation in order to reduce the rate of mechanical loosening; (2) Designing a better glenoid component to achieve the lowest possible rate of wear. But still the main cause of TSA failure has remained the aseptic loosening of the glenoid component [6].

2. Aseptic loosening

Aseptic loosening of endoprostheses occurs as a result of immune rejection response to an implanted foreign material. This response is enhanced when particles of polyethylene (from the glenoid insert), metal (from the glenoid metal backplate and/or from humeral component) or from fixating PMMA are released due to a mechanically abnormal gliding of the prosthesis. These particles, below 10μ in size, usually in $0.5\text{-}1.0\mu$ range [7], induce local and systemic recruitment of macrophages and osteoclasts [8], with subsequential generation of reactive pseudomembrane and local lysis of the prosthesis-bone interface [9] (Figure 1). The lysis of the fixation interface of the prosthesis causes its eventual loosening. Since in the TSA prosthesis the glenoid component is exposed to the higher stresses and usually constructed, at least partly, from polyethylene, it's loaded surface is prone to wear and its surrounding is exposed to the wear particles' seeding. For this reason the immune rejection response is concentrated mainly around the glenoid component.

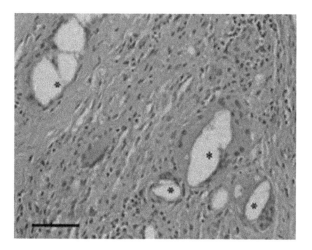

Figure 1. Micrograph (scale 200μ, HE staining) of pseodocapsule retrieved from the surface of a failed prosthesis. Characteristic foreign body reaction [10] is evident around areas of debris (*).

3. Mechanical considerations

The main cause of the wear of the glenoid component is its high loading by the eccentric forces. The excessive eccentric forces are generated when the transverse axis of the implanted glenoid is situated in a position which is incompatible with normal anatomical version of glenoid, e. g. between 2^0 of anteversion and 13^0 of retroversion [11]. This might happen when the prosthesis is implanted in an arthritic joint with advanced erosion of the posterior glenoid. Therefore care should be taken to reshape the glenoid towards an anteverted surface, in the physiological range, prior to implantation of the glenoid component [12].

In the longitudinal axis the excessive eccentric forces are generated when the superior stabilization of the humeral head is insufficient, therefore in patients with massive tears of the rotator cuff muscles an implantation of the glenoid component is contraindicated.

The full conformity between the TSA prosthesis components may also lead to an enhanced stress on the globoid rim due to the loss of the humeral head translation, which is possible in the normal shoulder joint, and as a consequence there is a higher risk for prosthetic loosening. [13,14]. The exact degree of optimal mismatch of the glenoid and the humeral head radii is not known. Furthermore the suboptimal mismatch of the glenoid and humeral component curvature can lead to a considerable rate of polyethylene wear due to an uneven force distribution between the components and a point loading and a point wear of the polyethylene [14].

4. Material considerations

There are several unique issues in TSA that should be addressed in the prosthesis design. First is a limited space and a limited bone stock for the glenoid component implantation. Two main difficulties arise due to this limitation:

1. The fixation area of the glenoid component is limited, either for cemented or cementless fixation. In order to increase fixation interface the glenoid components bear keels (central or in offset position), pegs (straight or tapered) and/or curved backsurface of the insert. It is not clear what type of fixation design is optimal for the cemented fixation [11]. There is some clinical evidence that a central tapered peg on a metal back-plate, covered by hydroxyapatite for enhanced ossiointegration, and initially fixed by two screws, might reduce loosening rate of glenoid component in cementless press fit fixation [15] (Figure 2).

2. The polyethylene gliding surface is essential in most designs of the glenoid component. The polyethylene surface should be at least 3 mm thick, preferably 4-6 mm thick, in order to diminish its wear following interaction with metal head of the humeral component [16]. This requirement prevents the versatile use of the cementless designs of a glenoid component, because they require the use of a metal back-plate under the polyethylene insert, with essential limitation of the later thickness in order to prevent the joint overstuffing. For this reason there is a high preference for use of all polyethylene made glenoid components for cemented implantation. This type of design allows the use of more thick polyethylene component, with lower wear rate. But the cemented fixation of this type of glenoid component might produce thermal mediated, adjacent to the implant, bone necrosis while PMMA polymerization and therefore eventually an enhanced loosening. Currently there is no clear information which of the fixation methods of the glenoid component is clinically advantageous.

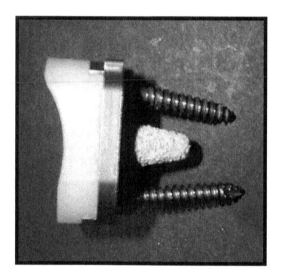

Figure 2. An example of glenoid component for cementless implantation: a polyethylene insert mounted on a metal back-plate with tapered peg covered by hydroxyapatite. The initial press fit fixation is enhanced by two screws. This design showed improved survivorship rates.

5. Clinical signs of the glenoid component loosening

The clinical signs of the TSA prosthesis failure include an increased level of pain during follow-up, that appeared to be related to the implant, with restriction of external rotation to under 20° and abduction to under 60° and/or newly developed radiolucency at the glenoid component interface with the underlying bone, more than 2mm in width [17]. The recognition of coexistence of both physical and radiographic signs is essential, since the isolated finding of periprosthetic radiolucency, without pain or significant restriction of movements of the shoulder, might not be of a high clinical importance (Figure 3). This consideration should be undertaken carefully in order to avoid unnecessary revision surgery. In all the cases of suspected TSA prosthesis loosening a standard workup for possible periprosthetic infection should be done in order to avoid a devastating misdiagnosis [18] (the discussion of this topic is out of the scope of the present chapter).

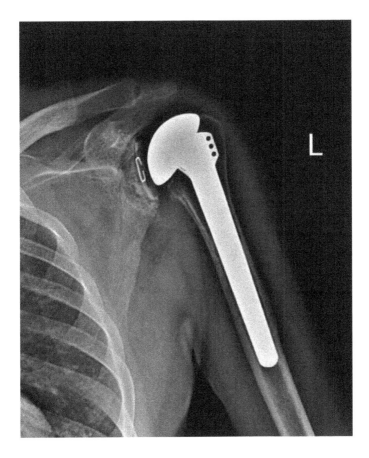

Figure 3. A shoulder radiograph (anterior-posterior view) of 60 years old male patient, three years after cemented TSA. Lucency is evident in the direct proximity to the glenoid component, but the patient is pain free and has good range of movements of the operated shoulder, without any laboratory evidence of infection and is satisfied from the function of the operated shoulder.

6. Survivorship data of TSA prostheses with special emphasis on glenoid loosening

In order to get a meaningful evaluation of the implanted prostheses longevity a powerful statistical tool of survivorship analysis is used [19]. Because the relative complicity in this method implementation, especially in defining the criteria for the "failure" of the implanted prostheses, only few reports on survivorship data of TSA exist, mainly with the parameter of a revision surgery as the indication of the failed prosthesis.

From the few reported survivorship data a short-term glenoid failure, requiring implant removal, reaches the rate of around 6% for cemented designs and 3% for cementless designs. Overall the glenoid component failure is the cause of between 20% - 60% of all failed TSAs, cemented or cementless (Table 1). Survivorship of TSA is the highest in patients with rheumatoid arthritis and the lowest in patients implanted following trauma and fracture. The reason is probably a lower demand for shoulder activity in the former group and expectations for nearly normal function in the latter group of patients [20, 21, 22, 23].

Reference	Type of prosthesis	No. of Patients	Survivorship	End point criteria	Glenoid failure rate	Overall failure rate
Tarchia et al [21]	Neer I & II cemented	113 [31=OA, 36=RA 12=2ary OA]	10years= 93% 15years= 87%	Revision – severe pain, abd<90°, ext rot<20°	7/113	14/113
Brenner et al [23]	Neer II & Gristina cemented	51 [37=OA 14=RA]	11years= 75%	Severe pain, radiographic evidence of component loosening	3/51	6/51
Cofield [22]	Cofield cementless	180 [110=OA 28=RA 30=2ary OA 12=revisions]	Not calculated	Revision	5/180	12/180
Pfahler et al [20]	Aequalis cemented	705 [418=OA 107=RA 180=2ary OA]	Not calculated	Revision	9/705	43/705

OA = osteoarthritis, RA = rheumatoid arthritis

Table 1. Long term survivorship data on cemented and the outcome of a large series of a cementless total shoulder replacement prostheses.

7. Treatment of loose glenoid

Surgical revision of failed glenoid should address several crucial factors. One of the main factors for consideration is the preservation of an adequate bone stock following the component removal. This is essential if replantation is considered, otherwise the component resection will be the definite procedure. Interestingly several authors reported that a resection of the failed glenoid component without subsequential replantation of a new component might cause a considerably favorable clinical outcome [24].

The second crucial factor is the preservation of adequate version of the remained glenoid in order to avoid future eccentric loads on the replanted glenoid component.

These two factors can be achieved by bone grafting, autologous or by allograft, with additional controlled reaming of the remained glenoid surface. The surgeon's arsenal of glenoid components for replantation includes parts for either cemented or cementless fixation, and biological soft tissue allografts for biological resurfacing. Several reports support the use of soft tissue allograft material, e.g. Achilles tendon, meniscus etc., for glenoid resurfacing in revision surgery [25]. Finally the replantation of the glenoid component might be immediate, during the revision surgery, or late, following initial bone grafting of cavitations and/ or bone deficiencies in the treated glenoid. Since this type of surgery has no standard guidelines because of the different patterns of the bone loss of the treated glenoids, a precise surgical protocol does not exist for this purpose and a lot of the decision making depends on the surgeon's experience and methodical preferences.

In order to avoid an extensive tissue damage during the glenoid revision surgery an arthroscopic approach has been suggested and reported in a small number of published reports. This method was popularized by O'Driscoll SW et al [26]. The authors used an arthroscopic approach through the standard anterior and posterior portals, with addition of another extended portal for the glenoid component remnants' retrieval. This method is suitable only for all-polyethylene components, because they should be cut in situ to at least 3 parts (by diagonal cuts using an inserted through the portal osteotom) in order to retrieve pieces in sizes which are compatible with the retrieval portal diameter. This method allows also a subsequential bone grafting of the exposed glenoid undersurface by using metal impactors which are inserted through the created portals [27]. This is a technically demanding technique, especially due to the optical interference, e.g. "mirror effect", that is caused by the metal humeral component head and due to the difficulty to control bleeding from the exposed glenoid surface. But because of the appealing tissue preservation this method might gain more widespread use in the future.

8. Prospective on the future improvement of the glenoid component design

Two main issues should be considered when seeking the improvement of the TSA survivorship. First of all the currently used TSA methods have already reached a high, above 90%, middle and long term survivorship rate, leaving a small, but important margin for improvement [21]. Secondary it is clear that this margin for improvement is related to the glenoid component design, since most of the failed TSAs are due to glenoid component failure. There is an example supporting this claim, when following a change of the design of the glenoid component a 10% increase in a short term survivorship of cementless TSA prosthesis has been achieved [15].

Clearly the main changes in the glenoid component design should address the rate of wear of this component and the efficiency of the component fixation. Therefore it is logical that the prospective for improvement of these issues will be related to finding the articulating surfaces generating less wear particles, even when subjected to excessive eccentric loading. Probably improving the biological osseous integration into the glenoid component will solve the complications of the current fixation either by the PMME or by the mechanical press fit fixation techniques. Some indications of the efficiency of biological fixation of the glenoid component have been already revealed in the devices coated by osteoconductive material, such as hydroxyapatite.

Author details

Nahum Rosenberg[1*], Maruan Haddad[2] and Doron Norman[2]

*Address all correspondence to: nahumrosenberg@Hotmail.Com

1 Rambam – Health Care Campus, Laboratory of Musculoskeletal Research, Department of Orthopaedic Surgery, Haifa, Israel

2 Rambam – Health Care Campus, Department of Orthopaedic Surgery. Haifa, Israel

References

[1] Neer CS: Replacement Arthroplasty for Glenohumeral Arthritis. J Bone Joint Surg Am 1974; 56-A113

[2] Brems J: The Glenoid Component in Total Shoulder Arthroplasty. J Shoulder Elbow Surg 1993; 2 47-54

[3] Crites BM, Berend ME, Ritter MA. Technical Considerations of Cemented Acetabular Components: a 30-year Evaluation. Clin Orthop 2000; 382 114-119

[4] Pfahler M, Jena F, Neyton L, Sirveaux F, Mole D, Cedex N: Hemiarthroplasty Versus Total Shoulder Prosthesis: Results of Cemented Glenoid Components. J Shoulder Elbow Surg 2006; 15 154-163.

[5] Tarchia ME, Cofield RH, Settergren CR . Total Shoulder Arthroplasty with the Neer Prosthesis: Long-Term Results. J Shoulder Elbow Surg 1997, 6:495-505.

[6] Hasan SS, Leith JM, Campbell B, Kapil R, Smith KL, Matsen FA. Characteristics of Unsatisfactory Shoulder Arthroplasties. J Shoulder Elbow Surg 2002; 11 431-41.

[7] Hallab NJ, Jacobs JJ. Biologic Effects of Implant Debris. Bul NYU Hosp Joint Dis 2009;67(2) 182-188

[8] Ren PG, Irani A, Huang Z, Ma T, Biswal S, Goodman SB. Continuous Infusion of UNMWPE Particles Induces Increased Bone Macrophages and Osteolysis. Clin Orthop Relat Res 2011; 469 113-122

[9] Purdue PE, Koulouvaris P, Nestor BJ, Sculco TP. The Central Role of Wear Debris In Periprosthetic Osteolysis. HSSJ 2006; 2 102-113

[10] Pandey R, Drakoulakis E, Athanasou NA. An Assessment of The Histological Criteria Used to Diagnose Infection in Hip Revision Artroplasty Tissue. J Clin Pathol 1999; 52 118-123

[11] Strauss EJ, Roche C, Flurin PH, Wright T, Zuckerman JD. The Glenoid In Shoulder Arthroplasty. J Shoulder Elbow Surg 2009; 18 819-833

[12] Farron A, Terrier A, Buchler P. Risks Of Loosening of a Prosthetic Glenoid Implanted In Retroversion. J Shoulder Elbow Surg 2006; 15 521-526

[13] Harryman DT, Sidles JA, Harris SL, Lippitt SB, Matsen FA. The Effect of Articular Conformity and the Size of the Humeral Head Component on Laxity and Motion after Glenohumeral Arthroplasty. J Bone Joint Surg Am 1995; 77-A 555-563

[14] Walch G, Edwards TB, Boulahia A, Boileau P, Mole D, Adeleine P. The Influence of Glenohumeral Prosthetic Mismatch on Glenoid Radiolucent Lines. Results of a multicenter study. J Bone Joint Surg Am 2002; 84-A 2186-2191.

[15] Rosenberg N, Neumann L Modi A, Mersich IJ, Wallace AW. Improvements In Survival of the Uncemented Nottingham Total Shoulder Prosthesis: A Prospective Comparative Study. BMC Musculoskeletal Disorders 2007; 8 76 - 87

[16] Brems J: The Glenoid Component In Total Shoulder Arthroplasty. J Shoulder Elbow Surg 1993; 2 47-54.

[17] Wallace AL, Walsh WR, Sonnabend DH: Dissociation of The Glenoid Component In Cementless Total Shoulder Arthroplasty. J Shoulder Elbow Surg 1999; 8 81-84

[18] Zimmerli W., Trampuz A., Ochsner PE. Prosthetic-joint Infections. N Engl J Med 2004; 351(16) 1645-1654

[19] Rosenberg N, Soudry M. Survivorship Analysis of Orthopaedc Procedures – Practical Approach. Arthroscopy 2011; 27(suppl 4) 16-24

[20] Pfahler M, Jena F, Neyton L, Sirveaux F, Mole D, Cedex N. Hemiarthroplasty Versus Total Shoulder Prosthesis: Results of Cemented Glenoid Components. J Shoulder Elbow Surg 2006; 15 154-163

[21] Tarchia ME, Cofield RH, Settergren CR . Total Shoulder Arthroplasty with the Neer Prosthesis: Long-Term Results. J Shoulder Elbow Surg 1997; 6 495-505

[22] Cofield RH: Uncemented Total Shoulder Arthroplasty. Clin Orthop 1994; 307 86-93

[23] Brenner BC, Ferlic DC, Clayton ML, Dennis DA. Survivorship of Unconstrained Total Shoulder Arthroplasty. J Bone Joint Surg Am 1989; 71-A 1289-1296

[24] Raphael BS, Dines JS, Warren RF , Figgie M, Craig EV. Symptomatic Glenoid Loosening Complicating Total Shoulder Arthroplasty. HSSJ 2010; 6 52 -56

[25] Namdari S, Gel DP, Wrner JJ. Managing Glenoid Bone Loss In Revision Total Shoulder Arthroplasty: A Review. UPOJ 2010; 20 44-49

[26] O'Driscoll SW, Petrie RS, Torchia ME. Arthroscopic Removal of the Glenoid Component for Failed Total Shoulder Arthroplasty. A Report of Five Cases. J Bone Joint Surg Am 2005; 87-A 858-863

[27] Namdari S, Glaser D. Arthroscopically Assisted Conversion of Total Shoulder Arthroplasty to Hemiarthroplasty with Glenoid Bone Grafting. Orthopedics 2011;34(11) 862-865

Periprosthetic Infection

Chapter 6

Peri-Prosthetic Joint Infection: Prevention, Diagnosis and Management

Adrian J. Cassar Gheiti and Kevin J. Mulhall

Additional information is available at the end of the chapter

1. Introduction

Total Joint Arthroplasty (TJA) is a safe and effective procedure that improves the quality of life and restores function in most patients suffering from joint arthritis. Post-operative peri-prosthetic joint infections (PJI) are an uncommon and difficult complication of joint replacement surgery.

PJI affects 1-3% total joint replacements and is the most common indication for revision in total knee arthroplasty (TKA) and third most common indication for revision total hip arthroplasty (THA)[1-4]. PJI can be difficult to diagnose and can present at any time from the primary procedure[5, 6]. PJI is painful, disabling, costly and often requires multiple procedures[7], prolonged periods of rehabilitation, antibiotic treatment and poor functional outcome. It places a considerable burden on hospital and surgeon resources with an estimated annual cost of infected revisions in US hospitals increasing from $320 million in 2001 to $566 million in 2009, with a projected cost exceeding $1.62 billion by 2020[8]. Consistent efforts at prevention are mandatory, and treatment of infection requires appropriate assessment of its chronicity and causative factors, the status of the wound and the overall health of the patient.

We will first provide an overview on peri-prosthetic joint infection and the possible risk factors involved. Finally, we will provide an overview of the current evidence available in preventing, diagnosis and managing peri-prosthetic joint infection.

2. Pathophysiology

Peri-prosthetic joint infections are a result of an intricate interaction between the host, the pathogen and the implant[9-11]. There is a multitude of host factors, ranging from medical comorbidities to social economic status, which increase the risk of PJI[9, 10, 12-15].

2.1. Host and environmental factors

Predisposing factors for PJI can be sub classified into preoperative, intraoperative and post-operative factors (Table 1). Preoperative predisposing factors include medical conditions such as diabetes, inflammatory arthropathies, preoperative anemia, congestive heart disease and chronic pulmonary disease to mention few[9, 10, 12, 14]. Intraoperative predisposing factors include simultaneous bilateral joint arthroplasty, longer operative time, knee arthroplasty, increased operating room traffic and contamination by the surgical team during preparation and draping[12, 16-19].

Post-operative predisposing factors to PJI include immunosuppressive medications, allogenic blood transfusion, post-operative atrial fibrillation, myocardial infarction, urinary tract infection and longer hospital stay[9, 10, 12].

Peri-prosthetic joint infections are typically caused by microorganisms that grow in biofilms[36]. Within biofilms, microorganisms in a polymetric matrix and develop into organized complex communities resembling a multicellular organism[37]. In a biofilm, microbes are protected from antimicrobial agents and host immune responses. This may be related to the reduced growth rate of biofilm microorganisms, which enter a stationary phase of growth[38]. Different microbes have different interactions with the host and the prosthetic. Some have specific adhesion molecules which help them adhere to the implant until a biofilm is formed, which is mediated in part by intracellular adhesion molecules[39]. Initially, adherent microorganisms and early biofilms are relatively unstable and still susceptible to host defense and antimicrobial agents. In contrast, mature biofilms are more stable and resist to elimination[40]. Furthermore, implants are devoid of microcirculation, which is crucial for the immune system and antibiotics to interact with microbes. Implants also tend to activate neutrophils which release peptides that deactivate granulocytes, impairing the removal of microbes[41]. This effect on granulocytes reduces the minimal amount of microbes that are required to cause an infection[41]. Inoculation of implants, not only occurs during the time of surgery, but can occur in the presence of a bacteremia from any source in the human body during the entire lifetime of the implant[42].

2.2. Microbial profile in PJI

A multitude of organisms mostly bacteria and fungi are reported to cause PJI (Table.2). The most reported organisms responsible for PJI are Gram positive *cocci*, most commonly *Staphylococcus Aureus* and *Staphylococcus Epidermidis* as reported by various authors[12, 20, 22, 31, 43-45]. On certain occasions, Gram negative bacteria and Fungi can also be responsible for periprosthetic joint infections[46, 47]. In a recent study published by Buller et al., Methicillin Resistant *Staph. Aureus* (MRSA) and Methicillin Resistant *Staph. Epidermidis* (MRSE) account for about 15.5% of all PJIs[20] and according to other studies up to 19% of PJIs can be poly microbial[12, 22, 48]. These microorganisms can all be part of normal skin flora; hence, direct inoculation at the time of the operation as well as airborne contamination are the most likely causes of these infections.

Predisposing Factors	Studies
Preoperative	
Male sex	Buller et al.[20], Jämsen et al.[21]
Socioeconomic status	Pulido et al.[12], Berbari et al.[22]
ASA > 2	Pulido et al.[12], Buller et al.[20], Bozic et al.[9], Saleh et al.[23],
Diabetes and elevated blood sugars	Buller et al.[20], Bozic et al.[9], Jämsen et al.[24], Berbari et al[22]., Saleh et al.[23]
Inflammatory Arthropathy	Pulido et al.[12], Bozic et al.[9], Wilson et al.[10], Jämsen et al.[21] , Berbari et al.[22]
Immunosuppressant medication	Wilson et al.[10], Berbari et al.[22], Saleh et al.[23]
Preoperative Anaemia	Pulido et al.[12], Greenky et al.[14], Bozic et al.[9]
Poor Nutrition	Berbari et al.[22]
Higher BMI	Pulido et al.[12], Bozic et al.[9]
Other infected Joint Arthroplasty	Buller et al.[20], Jafari et al.[15], Berbari et al.[22]
History of malignancy/metastasis	Bozic et al.[9], Berbari et al.[22]
Skin ulcers/PVD	Bozic et al.[9], Wilson et al.[10], Berbari et al.[22], Poss et al.[25]
Intraoperative	
Knee arthroplasty	Pulido et al.[12], Buller et al.[20]
Simultaneous bilateral	Pulido et al.[12]
Longer operative time	Pulido et al.[12], Muilwijk et al.[26], Ong et al.[27], Berbari et al.[22], Saleh et al.[23]
No prophylactic antibiotic	Fogelberg et al.[28], Pavel et al.[29], Meehan et al.[30], Al-Maiyah et al.[31]
Cement with no antibiotics	Hanssen AD.[32], Jämsen et al.[21]
Skin Preparation and Draping	Johnson et al.[33], Katthagen et al.[16]
Contamination by operating room personnel	Ayers et al.[34], Rao et al.[35]
Operating Room Traffic	Panahi et al.[18]
Postoperative	
Renal impairment	Pulido et al.[12], Saleh et al.[23], Bozic et al.[9]
Allogenic blood transfusion	Pulido et al.[12], Berbari et al.[22], Saleh et al.[23]
Myocardial Infarction	Pulido et al.[12]
Atrial fibrillation	Pulido et al.[12], Berbari et al.[22]
Urinary tract infection	Pulido et al.[12], Wilson et al.[10], Poss et al.[25]
Haematoma	Pulido et al.[12], Jämsen et al.[21], Berbari et al.[22], Saleh et al.[23]
Continuous wound discharge	Pulido et al.[12], Jämsen et al.[21], Berbari et al.[22]
Prolonged Hospital stay	Pulido et al,[12]. Berbari et al.[22]

Table 1. Predisposing factors to PJI

Organism	Study (number of cases)							
	Buller et al [342]	Mahmud et al [250]	Romano et al [71]	Pulido et al [63]	Berbari et al [462]	Phillips et al [75]	Al-Maiyah et al [106]	Salvati et al [2330]
Staphylococcus								
MRSA	13.5%	3.2%	31%	19%	22%	4%	6.6%	27.3%
MSSA	19.6%	16%	21.1%	19%		25%		
MRSE	2%	21.2%	22.5%	11%	19%	36%	68.9%	27.8%
MSSE	19.9%							
α-Hemolytic Streptococcus	3.8%							0.7%
β-Hemolytic Streptococcus	6.1%	2.8%	5.6%	12.7%	9%	7%		7.2%
γ-Hemolytic Streptococcus	4.1%							5.6%
Enterococcus	2.9%		5.6%	1.6%	1.2%	9%		4.5%
VRE	0.6%							
Streptococcus milleri	0.6%							
Peptostreptococcus	2.4%		2.8%				12.3%	
Gram-positive rods								
Corynebacterium	0.3%		1.4%	1.6%	0.6%			3.2%
Enterobacter	4.1%	1.6%						1%
Propionibacterium	2.9%	0.8%	2.8%			1%		1.7%
Gram negative								
Escherichia coli	3.2%	1.2%		3.2%		4%	0.9%	5.5%
Haemophilus	0.3%							
Citrobacter koseri	0.3%							0.1%
Klebsiella	1.2%			3.2%		3%		1.3%
Proteus mirabilis	2.0%			1.6%				3.1%
Pseudomonas	3.2%	0.8%	5.6%	1.6%		4%	1.9%	5.6%
Salmonella	0.9%					1%		0.3%
Serratia marcescens	0.3%	1.2%	1.4%	1.6%				0.3%
Bacteroides fragilis	0.3%	0.4%						0.5%
Yeasts								
Candida	0.3%				0.2%			0.3%
Diphteroids						1%	9.4%	0.9%
Polymicrobial		0.02%		6.3%	19%			
Culture negative	8.8%	27.2%		9.5%	12%			
No Results		22.4%						

MRSA: Methicillin Resistant *Staph. aureus*, MSSA: Methicillin Sensitive *Staph. aureus,* MRSE: Methicillin Resistant *Staph. epidermis*. MSSE: Methicillin Sensitive *Staph. epidermis*.

Table 2. Percentage of microbes in PJI [12, 20, 22, 31, 43-45, 48]

While, the patient's endogenous flora is largely held accountable for surgical site infections, the surgical team personnel and operating room environment may also contribute to disperse organisms[49] and increase the bacterial count[18, 50]. Members of the surgical team who have direct contact with sterile field have been linked to outbreaks of unusual organism such as *Serratia Marcescens*[51]. Even though anesthesiologists, are not directly involved in the operative field, they perform a variety of procedures related to the operation and have been associated with outbreaks of bloodstream and surgical site infections linked to the reuse of propofol vials and other deviations from acceptable protocols[52].

2.3. Classification of PJI

The classification of PJI is based on, either the type of pathogenesis or the time of clinical manifestation. When PJI are classified according to the pathogenesis, inoculation of the surgical site occurs either exogenously or haematogenously[11]. Exogenous infection, are infections that occur during surgery or in the early post-operative period, usually in the presence of large hematomas. Haematogenous infections are acquired through the bloodstream at any time after surgery. As discussed in section 2.1, it has been reported that implants impair the immune defenses and decrease the minimal abscess-forming dose of *Staph. aureus* at least 10 000 fold both in an animal and human model[53, 54]. Patients with prosthetic joints have a reported risk of 30 - 40% for haematogenous device–associated infection during *Staph. aureus* sepsis[13, 42]. Even though patients, are mostly susceptible to PJI early after implantation, haematogenous infection can occur at any time after surgery.

More commonly, PJI is classified according to the time of clinical manifestation after total joint replacement. This classification is divided into 4 stages or groups[11, 55, 56]:

• Stage I or Early post-operative infection, which present acutely within the first 4 to 8 weeks after the operation

• Stage II or Delayed onset PJI and occurs between the 3rd month up to 24 months after surgery

• Stage III or Late onset PJI usually occur after 2 years from the procedure, the presentation is usually sudden in an otherwise well-functioning joint.

• Stage IV or Silent infection when a positive culture is found at time of revision without any previous evidence of infection.

Early (Stage I), delayed (Stage II) and silent (Stage IV) infections are commonly exogenous, while stage I infections are probably caused by virulent microorganisms such as *Staph. aureus* and *Escherichia coli*, Stage II and Stage IV are typically caused by low virulent bacteria such as coagulase negative staphylococci and *Propionbacterium acnes[56, 57]*. Stage III or Late onset PJI occur acutely in a well-functioning joint and are caused by haematogenous spread. The most common primary focus of infection is from skin and soft tissue infections, but seeding from urinary, respiratory, gastrointestinal tract and dental infections are also reported[58]. In a recent report by Sendi et al., 57.5% of cases with haematogenous PJI had no source identified either because of primary bacteremia, or because the primary infection has already healed by the time signs and symptoms of PJI present[13].

2.4. Definition of PJI

The Musculoskeletal Infection Society (MSIS) have recently analyzed the available evidenced and proposed a set of criteria to define peri-prosthetic joint infection.

Based on these criteria[59], a definite PJI exists when:

i.   there is a sinus tract communicating with the prosthesis; or

ii.   a pathogen is isolated by culture from 2 or more separate tissue or fluid samples obtained from the affected prosthetic joint; or

iii.   when 4 of the following 6 criteria exist;

   a.   elevated serum erythrocyte sedimentation rate and serum C-reactive protein (CRP) concentration,

   b.   elevated synovial white blood cell count,

   c.   elevated synovial polymorphonuclear percentage(PMN%),

   d.   presence of purulence in the affected joint

   e.   isolation of a microorganism in one culture of periprosthetic tissue or fluid, or

   f.   greater than 5 neutrophils per high-power field in 5 high-power fields observed from histologic analysis of periprosthetic tissue at ×400magnification.

PJI may be present if less than 4 of these criteria re not met and that in certain infections with low virulent organisms such as *Propionibacetium acnes,* several of these criteria may not be routinely met despite the presence of PJI.

3. Prevention of PJI

Both the host and environmental factors described previously (Table. 1) can affect the risk for developing PJI. An effective strategy in preventing PJI is to improve both host and environmental factors during the pre, intra and post-operative period (Table. 3).

There are a number of host factors that increase the risk of PJI including conditions such as diabetes, inflammatory arthropathy, preoperative anaemia, poor nutrition and obesity to mention a few(Table. 1). Patients who present for elective orthopaedics procedures are in suboptimal health. Furthermore, the impact of various risk factors appears to be accumulative, such that each factor has an individual affect to increase the risk of infection and has a synergistic potential on the risk conferred by other factors[60, 61]. Thus, identifying such risk factors and addressing them in the preoperative setting is critical in reducing PJI and other postoperative complication.

Time			Strategy
Preoperative	Early	Host optimization	Improve Diabetic control
			Treat possible site of infections
			Improve possible Medical Comorbidities
			Obesity + Improve Nutritional Status
			Pre – operative anaemia
			Smoke Cessation
			MRSA screening
	Day of Surgery	Surgical Site Optimization	Surgical Site Shaving
			Skin decolonisation (CHG wipes/showers)
Intraoperative		Surgical factors	Prophylactic antibiotics
			Skin Preparation
			Draping
			Bleeding Control
			Antibiotic impregnated cement
			Skin Closure
			Wound Dressing
		Surgical team	Decolonization: Surgical scrubbing/rubbing
			Impermeable Gowns/PPS
			Double Gloving
		OR environment	Operating Room Traffic
			Laminar Airflow
Post-operative		Immediate	Antibiotics for 24 hours
			Wound management
			Blood Transfusion only where indicated
			Management of medical complications
		Late	Antibiotic prophylaxis before invasive procedures

CHG: Chlorhexadine Gluconate, OR: Operating Room, PPS: Personal Protection System, MRSA: Methicillin Resistant Staph. aureus Adopted from Matar et al. Preventing infection in total joint arthroplasty. J Bone Joint Surg Am. 2010;92 Suppl 2:36-46. Epub 2010/12/09.

Table 3. Preoperative, Intraoperative and Post-operative Strategies in preventing PJI

3.1. Pre-operative period

3.1.1. Health optimization

Pre-operative optimization of health is of crucial importance to ensure a satisfactory outcome following total joint arthroplasty. ASA scores >2, diabetes and rheumatoid arthritis among several factors have been associated with increased rates of perioperative complications and PJI after total joint arthroplasty[9, 12, 20, 21, 24]. Lei et al. and Malinzak et al. have both reported that diabetes and the total number of comorbidities were associated with a higher risk of infection and that medical conditions have a synergistic effect on the risk of developing a PJI[60, 62].

Prior to total joint arthroplasty, all patients should be assessed and managed in a multidisciplinary pre-assessment clinic to optimize their general health. These have been shown to significantly reduce both the post-operative mortality and costs per admission in orthopaedic surgery[63]. Pre Assessment Clinics (PAC), focus on optimizing the host health in the preoperative period such as improving nutritional status, optimizing diabetic control, cardiac and respiratory comorbidities and screening for possible source of infection and MRSA decolonization. In our institution, all patients are assessed in the pre assessment clinic by a consultant anesthesiologist, specialist nurse, nutritionist and physiotherapist, and if necessary further consultation with other medical specialists such as cardiologist, rheumatologist or neurologists is available to optimize the patients' health preoperatively. The anesthetic consultant also follows the patient during hospitalization and during the post-operative period whenever possible.

3.1.2. Bacterial decolonization

The Centre for Disease Control (CDC) guidelines for prevention of surgical site infection (SSIs) has strongly recommended that patients require to shower or bathe with an antiseptic agent on at least the night before the operative day in order to reduce bacterial load[64]. While whole body bathing with antiseptic has been shown to reduce bacterial load of the skin as well as reducing the risk of infections[35, 65-67], it presents challenges in achieving entire body coverage and in maintaining sufficiently high concentrations of solution on the skin for effective antisepsis[68]. Further more patient compliance with these protocols is an issue[69]. Recent studies have addressed the effectiveness of preoperative protocols with chlorhexidine gluconate (CHG) applied twice daily by patients at home before their joint replacement[33, 70] and one study reported reduction in SSI infection from 3.19% to 1.59% after the introduction of 2% CHG in place of povidone iodine antiseptic[71]. Based on the results of these studies, home skin preparation seems to be a simple and cost effective technique in reducing PJI but patient compliance is an issue and further randomized control trials are required to fully understand the effect on preventing PJI.

3.1.3. Prophylactic antibiotics

The benefits of prophylactic antibiotics have been widely reported in orthopaedic literature [28-30, 72]. In 1970, Foldberg et al. compared a group treated prophylactically with penicillin given preoperatively, intraoperatively and up to 5 days post operatively, with a control group not treated with antibiotics; both groups underwent a mixture of mold arthroplasties and spinal fusions[28]. The prevalence of infections was 1.7% in the treated group while 8.9% in the control group[28]. Furthermore during the period of the study these authors have noticed an increase in the prevalence of MRSA in all major orthopaedic wound infections, which demonstrates a delicate balance between the use and overuse of antibiotics in the prevention and treatment of infections.

The most common organisms responsible for PJI have been already discussed in section 2.2, and prophylactic antibiotics are targeted to cover this spectrum of organisms. Cefazolin and cefuroxamine are the antibiotics of choice because of their good tissue penetration and excellent activity against Staphylococci and Streptococci. The American Association of Orthopaedic Surgeons (AAOS) published guidelines regarding prophylactic choice, dosing and optimal postoperative duration[61]. The AAOS recommendations for the use of intravenous antibiotic prophylaxis are as follows:

- **Recommendation 1:** The antibiotic used for prophylaxis should be selected carefully, consistent with current recommendations in the literature, taking into account the issue of resistance and *patient allergies*. Currently, cefazolin and cefuroxamine are the preferred antibiotics for patients undergoing orthopaedic procedures. Clindamycin and vancomycin may be used in patients with known β-lactam allergy. Vancomycin may be used in patients with known colonization with MRSA or in facilities with recent MRSA outbreaks. In multiple studies, exposure to vancomycin is reported as a risk in the development of vancomycin resistant enterococcus (VRE) colonization and infection. Vancomycin should be reserved fir the treatment of serious infection with β-lactam resistant organisms or for treatment of infection in patients with life threatening allergy to β-lactam antimicrobials.

- **Recommendation 2:** Timing and dosage of antibiotics administration should optimize the *efficiency of the therapy*. Prophylactic antibiotics should be administered within 1 hour before skin incision. Owing to an extended infusion time, vancomycin should be started within 2 hours before incision. If a proximal tourniquet is used, the antibiotic must be completely infused before the inflation of the tourniquet. Dose amount should be proportional to the patients' weight; for patients who weigh more than 80Kg, Cefazolin dose should be doubled. Additional intraoperative doses of antibiotics are advised is [1] the duration of the procedure exceeds one to two tines the antibiotic's half-life or [2] there is significant blood loss during the procedure. The general guidelines for frequency of intraoperative antibiotic administration are as follows: cefazolin every 2-5 hours, cefuroxamine every 2-4 hours, clindamycin every 2-6 hours and vancomycin every 6-12 hours.

- **Recommendation 3:** Duration of prophylactic antibiotic administration should not exceed *the 24 hour postoperative period*. Prophylactic antibiotics should be discontinued within 24 hours of the end of surgery. The medical literature does not support the continuation of antibiotics until all drains or catheters are removed and provides no evidence of benefit when they are continued past the 24 hours.

3.2. Intra-operative period

3.2.1. Pre-operative hair removal

Pre-operative hair removal is of common practice, and a meta-analysis by the Cochrane group showed that the relative risk of surgical site infection following hair removal with a razor was significantly higher than that following hair removal with clippers, but there was no difference reported in the rate of post-operative infections between procedures preceded by hair removal and those performed without hair removal[73]. It is recommended that whenever hair is removed clippers rather than a razor should be used at the time of surgery[73].

3.2.2. Pre-operative skin preparation

3.2.2.1. Patients

Three main types of skin antiseptic agents are used; mainly chlorohexidine gluconate (CHG), alcohol based solutions and povidone-iodine. Chlorohexidine is favored due to its long lasting and cumulative activity against gram-positive and gram negative organisms found on human flora. Povidone iodine it is also effective in reducing skin flora but in becomes ineffective on contact with blood and duration of activity is shorter the CHG. Alcohol is an excellent antimicrobial but its effectiveness is limited by the lack of any residual activity after drying and the risk of flammability. A Cochrane meta-analysis carried out in 2004 showed no difference in efficiency among skin antiseptics used in clean surgery[74]. Recent studies strongly suggest that CHG combined with alcohol is superior to povidone-iodine combined with alcohol in antisepsis for patients[75-77]. Ostrander et al. reported reduced bacterial count on feet prepared with Chloraprep (2% CHG and 70% isopropyl alcohol; Medi-Flex, Overland Park, Kansas) than on those prepared with Duraprep (0.7% iodin and 74% isopropyl alcohol; 3M Healthcare, St. Paul, Minnesota) or Techni-Care[3.0% chloroxylenol; Care-Tech Laboratories, St. Louis, Missouri) but there was no difference in infection rates among the 3 groups[77].

3.2.2.2. Surgeon

Antiseptic agents for surgeons can be classified into hand scrubs agents and hand rub agents. Hand scrubs are typically solutions of CHG or povidone-iodine while hand rubs are typically alcohol based solutions. Most data indicates that povidone–iodine and CHG have equal efficacy in decreasing bacterial colony forming units from the skin of surgeons; furthermore no difference was found between hand rubs and hand scrub solutions[78, 79]. Some studies report better cost effectiveness of alcoholic hand rub by saving on water consumption and better physician compliance [78].

3.2.3. Draping

There is strong evidence in the literature for the use of plastic surgical adhesive tapes and nonpermeable paper drapes for surgical site draping [16, 80-83]. Nonpermeable drapes are used to prevent bacterial penetration during surgery, which was found to increase when traditional cloth drapes got wet[80]. Iobhan iodophor-impregnated drapes (3M Health Care) have been shown a reduction in wound contamination without any decrease in wound infection rate after total joint arthroplasty[84]. In their review of 4 000 patients in seven different trials, the Cochrane Wounds Group, found no evidence that adhesive drapes (plain or impregnated with antimicrobials) reduce surgical site infection rates[85].

3.2.4. Double gloving

Sterile surgical gloves aim to protect the patient from contamination from residual bacteria from members of the surgical team after hand scrubbing and protect the surgical team from the patient's body fluids[86]. Double gloving has been recommended because it has been shown that it reduces perforations in the innermost glove especially in orthopaedic procedures where sharp surfaces are easily formed[86-88]. Beldame et al. have reported that, 80% of glove perforations occur during surgical incision and changing the outer glove after surgical incision and before implantation of the prosthesis can reduce the risk of contamination and perforation and resulted in a sterile state in 80% of cases[89].

3.2.5. Laminar flow, operating room traffic and personal protection system

Operating theatres are designed to reduce bacterial exposure to patients during surgery. Vertical laminar airflow (LAF) provides directional airflow through a higher efficiency particulate air (HEPA) filters and positive air pressure within the surgical field. Multiple studies have reported reduced PJI rates with LAF[17, 90-92]. Brandt et al. reported no benefit from using LAF, and it was even associated with increased risk of surgical site infection after total hip arthroplasty. A recent systematic review on SSI following hip and knee arthroplasty included 8 studies over the past 10 years and showed no improvement on PJI rates and recommends against the installation of LAF systems in new operating theatres[93].

The opening of the operating room door disrupts the laminar airflow, allowing pathogens to enter the space surrounding the site of the operation with increased risk of PJI[17, 94, 95]. Panahi et al. have reported a mean rate of 0.69 door opening per minute for primary and 0.84 openings per minute for revision total joint arthroplasty. Only 8% of the traffic was determined to be due to scrubbing in and out, demonstrating a high rate of unjustifiable traffic, the authors further advise to implement strategies in reducing operating room traffic in an attempt to decrease one etiology of PJI[18].

The human exhaust system or personal protection system (PPS) was initially introduced by Sir J Charnley in the 1960s and designed to decrease airborne bacteria and intraoperative contamination in total joint arthroplasty[96]. No uniform opinion exists with regard to the use of PPS and the incidence of PJI[97-101]. One of the main issues with PPS is that, they are bulky and tend to get contaminated. In a recent study, Kearns et al. have reported that 53 out of 102 PPS tested were contaminated with staphylococcus and one with MRSA, which means that the PPS does not remain externally sterile in half of the cases[19]. These authors recommend refraining from touching the PPS during surgery and the need to change gloves if hand contact with the PPS occurs[19].

3.2.6. Operative time

Long operative times have been found to increase the risk for PJI after total joint arthroplasty[27, 102, 103]. From a cohort of 9245 patients undergoing total joint arthroplasty, Pulido et
al reported longer operative time as a predisposing factor for PJI, a finding which is also
supported Kurtz et al. and Peersman et al[104, 105]. Furthermore, surgeons volume seems to
be inversely proportional to the rate of infection, were the higher the surgeon volume the
lower the rate of infection, but this was only found to be statistically significant after total
knee arthroplasty[26].

3.2.7. Addition of antibiotics to cement

In recent years antibiotic impregnated cement has become a standard for use in cemented
primary arthroplasty. According to recent studies, the rate of PJI was lower when a combination of intravenous antibiotic prophylaxis and antibiotic impregnated cement was used
for primary cemented arthroplasty[21, 106]. Antibiotic impregnated cement seems to be of
particular use in the revision setting[107-109]. Nevertheless there is strong evidence to support the efficiency of combined regime of prophylactic antibiotic and cement impregnated
antibiotic when compared to prophylactic antibiotic only in patients with other risk factors
for PJI[32, 110, 111].

3.2.8. Wound closure and surgical dressing

Various methods of skin closure are used in arthroplasty surgery, ranging from skin staples,
subcuticular closure with absorbable suture and recently the use of knotless barbed sutures.
A recent meta-analysis by Smith et al. reported that closure with skin staples had a significant risk of wound infection when compared to traditional suturing, but out of the six studies reviewed only one study had acceptable methodology[112]. Newman et al has reviewed
181 patients after total knee arthroplasty and reported significant fewer complications after
closure with skin staples when compared with absorbable subcuticular sutures[113]. A prospective randomized control trial comparing staples to subcuticular absorbable suture and
tissue adhesives after TKA, showed highest superficial infection rate for subcuticular suture
(26%) and the lowest for skin staples (5%), although none of them required any treatment
with antibiotics[114]. Furthermore, staple based wound closure was fastest and the least expensive after TKA but had the longest hospital stay when compared to the other methods[114]. Recently there has been increased interest in knotless barbed sutures for wound
closure after total joint arthroplasty[115-117]. Most studies reported faster closure times for
the barbed sutures when compared to traditional methods[116, 117]. Patell et al. have reported a significant increase risk of major wound complications especially after TKA, when
barbed sutures (4.3%) were used compared to staples 1.1% and standard absorbable subcuticular closure (4.2%)[115]. However, debate still exists on which is the optimal method of
closure.

Surgical technique with careful tissue handling and wound closure is important in wound
healing, as well as the type of dressing that is applied postoperatively[118, 119]. Wound

dressing assist with healing by acting as a physical barrier to bacteria, splinting the wound to protect it from subsequent injury, helping with haemostasis, reducing dead space and minimizing pain. The use of occlusive dressings is well known to improve re-epithelisation and subsequent collagen synthesis when compared to wound exposed to air[120, 121]. In a recent Cochrane review, Dumville et al. reported no evidence to suggest that one dressing is better than any other in preventing surgical site infection and advised that the choice of dressing should be based on costs and the need for management of specific symptoms[122]. After total joint arthroplasty, a hydrofiber/hydrocolloid dressing using the jubilee method has been shown to reduce the rate of blister formation but no significant reduction in surgical site infection[118]. Burke et al. have carried out a prospective randomized study comparing the jubilee dressing method with standard adhesive dressing after total joint arthroplasty and reported a significant reduction in blister formation, leakage and dressing changes in the group treated with the jubilee method but no significant reduction in SSI. The authors of this study recommend the use of the hydrofiber/hydrocolloid dressing combination after total joint arthroplasty due to the associated lower complication rate[123].

3.3. Post-operative period

Most medical complications in the post-operative period have been to increased rates of PJI, mainly elevated blood creatinine levels, allogenic blood transfusion, myocardial infarction, atrial fibrillation and urinary tract infections[9, 10, 12, 21, 22, 25]. Adequate hydration is critical in post-operative period and allogenic blood transfusion is indicated in the presence of symptomatic anaemia, a haemoglobin level <8g/dL, or when it is medically indicated[124]. Control and monitoring of blood sugar levels is important in diabetic patients and should follow the same principles used in the preoperative period. Persistent wound drainage has been has been found as a contributing factor in the development of PJI[12, 21, 22], however there is little or no supportive evidence for the continues use of antibiotics[61] or antimicrobial impregnated dressings[122]. Furthermore, post-operative complication can result in delayed rehabilitation after a total joint arthroplasty with resultant delay in discharge from hospital, which has been reported by various studies as a risk factor for the development of PJI[12, 22].

4. Diagnosing PJI

Currently there is no diagnostic modality, which is 100% reliable in diagnosis PJI. An assessment using a combination of clinical findings and investigations is necessary.

4.1. Clinical

A careful history and physical examination are crucial in making a diagnosis of PJI. Although the diagnosis of early postoperative or acute haematogenous infection is not difficult, late infections can be challenging to distinguish from other causes of pain in a patient with previous total joint arthroplasty. Clinically, early or acute infections are characterized by pain, fever, wound drainage or erythema. While the only feature of chronic infection, can be pain unrelieved by a seemingly well-functioning arthroplasty. Loosening during the first year post implantation or a consistently painful arthroplasty should be considered infected until proven otherwise.

4.2. Diagnostic investigations

4.2.1. Serology

Erythrocyte Sedimentation Rate (ESR) and C-Reactive Protein (CRP) are baseline screening tests for any patient planned for revision arthroplasty regardless of the cause of failure[5]. Diagnostic value of ESR and CRP has been widely reported, and their combined use is a very good 'rule out' test [125, 126]. When both ESR and CRP are negative, periprosthetic infection is unlikely, however when both tests are positive PJI must be considered, and this warrants further investigations [5]. Ghanem et al. have reported that values higher than an ESR of 30 mm/h and CRP 10 mg/l combined to gather had 97.6% sensitivity for a positive diagnosis of PJI[127].

A full blood count including a white blood cell (WBC) count is part of the routine workout for patients with suspected PJI, however recent evidence suggests that serum WBC and differential carries a very low sensitivity (55% and 52% respectively) and specificity (66% and 75% respectively)[128]. Accordingly, routine serum WBC count and differential have no role in the diagnosis of PJI..

4.2.2. Joint aspiration

Joint aspiration is recommended as part of the work up in diagnosing PJI in patients with combined elevation of ESR and CRP levels in the hip and elevation of ESR and/or CRP levels in the knee joint[5]. Joint aspiration is usually carried out under sterile conditions, and synovial fluid should be for culture and sensitivity, WBC count and neutrophil percentage. Some patients with abnormal ESR and CRP may require more than one aspiration. A WBC count higher than 1700 cell/µl or a neutrophil percentage greater than 65% is highly suggestive of chronic PJI, however these values are not applicable when diagnosis acute PJI[129, 130]

4.2.3. Imaging studies

Imaging studies such as plain radiographs, computed tomography (CT) or magnetic resonance imaging (MRI) scans are useful in sub classifying patient into high and low probability of PJI. Radiolucent lines, focal osteolysis, periosteal bone formation or early loosening may all suggest PJI[131], however differentiating between PJI and aseptic loosening may not be possible using imaging modalities on their own. Nuclear scintigraphy detects inflammation in peri-prosthetic tissue, and although technetium-99m bone scintigraphy has very high sensitivity, it lacks specificity for infection[132]. A technetium bone scan can remain positive more than a year after implantation because of increased periprosthetic bone remodelling.

Love et al. reported increased sensitivity (96%), specificity (87%) and accuracy (91%) when a leukocyte/marrow scintigraphy was used to identify PJI. The test was significantly more accurate than bone (50%), bone/gallium (66%) and leuckocyte/bone (70%) scintigraphy in diagnosing PJI[133]. It seems that a Leukocyte/marrow scintigraphy will remain the procedure of choice in diagnosing PJI until agents capable of differentiating infection from aseptic inflammation are developed[133].

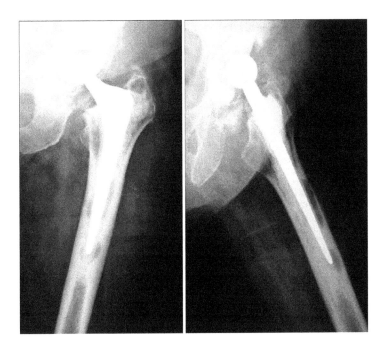

Figure 1. Plain AnteroPosterior and Lateral Radiographs showing focal areas of osteolysis, suspicious of PJI.

4.2.4. Intraoperative techniques

Various techniques can be used intraoperatively during revision arthroplasty to diagnose infection. These techniques include synovial fluid biomarkers, cultures and frozen sections.

4.2.4.1. Cultures and Gram stain

Cultures of periprosthetic tissues provide the most reliable means of detecting that pathogen and are often used as a reference standard in diagnosing PJI. Multiple samples should be taken at the time of the procedure from various regions, at least 3 samples for culture are recommended[134-136]. Cultures may be negative because prior antibiotic exposure, low number of organisms, an inappropriate culture medium, fastidious organisms or prolonged transport time to the laboratory[11]. Grams stains have high specificity (97%) but extreme low sensitivity (less than 26%)[137, 138]. The AAOS guidelines recommend against the routine use of intraoperative gram stain for the diagnosis of PJI[5].

4.2.4.2. Frozen sections

A meta-analysis by Della Valle et al reported that frozen sections are very good in ruling in but have low value in ruling out and infection[5]. These studies have more than 80% sensitivity and more than 90% specificity, but they also have high interobserver variability. The degree of inflammatory cells infiltrations varies among specimens from the same patient, sometimes even within individual tissue samples[11].

4.2.4.3. Synovial fluid biomarkers

Synovial fluid can used to analyse for various biomarkers such as leukocyte esterase, synovial CRP and white blood cell count, interleukin 6 (IL-6) and interleukin 8 (IL-8). Leukocyte esterase is an enzyme secreted by activated neutrophils that migrate at the site of infections. This enzyme is usually found on colorimetric dipsticks to diagnose urinary tract infections. Potential advantages of this diagnostic tool include wide availability, low cost and potential of an accurate diagnosis within minutes. Parvizi et al. have initially reported preliminary data on using leukocyte esterase as a diagnostic tool. These authors reported 80.6% sensitivity and 100% specificity in diagnosing PJI, with 100% positive predictive value and 93.3% negative predictive value[139]. Wetters et al also reported similar results when they used leukocyte esterase for diagnosis PJI[140]. In both studies, the leukocyte esterase strip was unreadable in on third off cases due to synovial blood or debris. Even though, these results are promising, both of these studies have their limitations in the methodology used, and further on, none of studies identifies whether the leukocyte esterase strip is able to differentiate between inflammation and infection.

Measurement of synovial CRP has been shown to be a sensitive (85%) and specific (95%) marker in diagnosis PJI[141, 142]. Recent studies report IL-6 levels to be more accurate in diagnosis PJI than ESR, CRP level, or synovial fluid WBC count and can be useful in diagnosis of PJI in patients with confounding systemic variables. Jacovides et al. have also reported higher specificity and sensitivity for both IL-6 (100% and 87.1%) and IL-8 (97.7% and 90.3%) when compared to synovial CRP (97.7% and 87.1%)[143]. Based on these studies synovial fluid biomarkers could provide an additional valuable resource for the diagnosis of PJI, but further studies are required.

4.3. AAOS guidelines

The American Academy of Orthopaedic Surgeons (AAOS), based on the current clinical evidence, has proposed clinical guidelines in the diagnosis of peri-prosthetic joint infection[144]. On the bases of the clinical features, the patients are classified into those who have a high or low probability of PJI (Table 4). The guidelines consist of 15 recommendations, with the majority being supported strongly in the literature. The guidelines advocate an algorithmic approach to the diagnosis of PJI, beginning with baseline investigations such the Erythrocyte Sedimentation Rate (ESR) and the C Reactive Protein (CRP) that carry high sensitivity and specificity when combined together[125, 126].

	One or more symptoms, AND at least one or more:
Higher Probability of Infection	• risk factor* OR
	• physical exam finding; OR
	• early implant loosening/osteolysis (as detected by x-ray)
	Pain or joint stiffness only and none of the following:
Lower Probability of Infection	• risk factors;* OR
	• physical exam findings; OR
	• early implant loosening/osteolysis (as detected by x-ray)

*risk factor supported by evidence or expert opinion. Adopted from the AAOS clinical practice guidelines for the diagnosis of periprosthetic infections[144]

Table 4. Stratification of patients into High or low probability of infection[144]

Further investigations, such as joint aspiration, are recommended in a stepwise manner depending on the ESR and CRP levels. The AAOS clinical guidelines and algorithms for the diagnosis peri-prosthetic infections, are available free to download from http://www.aaos.org/research/guidelines/guide.asp.

5. Management of PJI

The management of total joint arthroplasty consists of one or more of the following techniques:

i.   Antibiotic therapy

ii.   Debridement and Irrigation of the joint with component retention or linear exchange

iii.   Single Stage Revision Arthroplasty (SSRA)

iv.   Two Stage Revision Arthroplasty (TSRA)

v.   Arthrodesis

vi.   Amputation

Management decisions are made on severity, chronicity of the infection, virulence of the infecting organism, status of surrounding soft tissue and physiological status of the patient.

5.1. Unexpected positive intraoperative cultures

Unexpected positive intraoperative cultures are found in cases where pre-operative assessment fails to show infection, these cases usually undergo revision for aseptic loosening. Tsukayama eta al. reported up to 11% of cases were infection was diagnosed with positive intraoperative cultures and were all treated with 6 weeks of antibiotics without additional operation. Antibiotic therapy failed in 3 of these cases, and the patients required further surgical treatment with 2 patient showing evidence of recurrent infection at 2 year follow up[56]. In another study, 15 patients with positive intraoperative cultures were not treated with antibiotics, recurrence of infection was reported in 6 patients[145]. Based on these studies, patients with unexpected positive cultures should be treated with antibiotics for 6 weeks while monitoring their ESR and CRP values to assess response to treatment under the supervision of a specialist microbiologist[146].

5.2. Antibiotic suppression

When patients have poor state of health, have a high risk of complications after surgery and the infective organism is of low virulence and susceptible to antibiotic therapy, suppression by antibiotic alone may be the best option. Rao et al. investigated the rates of eradication of antibiotic resistant organisms with suppression therapy and noted eradication in 86% at mean follow up of five years, with five recurrent infections all within the first 3 years[147]. Antibiotic suppression is also indicated in patient with persistent PJI following surgical intervention if they decline or cannot tolerate further surgery[6, 11, 148, 149]. The literature on antibiotic suppressive therapy without any surgical intervention is poor; despite this, patients who cannot tolerate surgery have no other option than suppressive therapy.

5.3. Debridement and Irrigation with component retention or linear exchange

Operative debridement and irrigation with component retention should be reserved of acute infections (Stage II and occasionally stage III). Early infections may range in severity from superficial cellulitis to deep infections. Superficial infections associated with wound dehiscence or purulent drainage and infections with wound necrosis or infected haematomas often require surgical debridement. Reported eradication rate has been between 24% to 71 % following open debridement and irrigation[56, 150, 151]. Even though, some case reports show excellent results from irrigation and debridement[152], a recent multicentre retrospective study showed that irrigation and debridement with component retention is not affected by organism type and that this technique had a failure rate as high as 70%, with the authors questioning the actual role of irrigation and debridement in the treatment of PJI[151]. Prostheses retention is also contraindicated in those with multiple joint arthroplasty or when the duration of symptoms is more than 1 month[7, 15].

5.4. Single stage revision arthroplasty

Single stage revision with removal of components, debridement, irrigation and reimplantation of new components provides removal of infected prosthesis while limiting the number of surgeries, recovery time and costs. Callaghan et al. reports 8.3% rate of recurrence after single stage revision arthroplasty with a minimum follow up of 10 years[153]. The local therapy, is achieved by adding antibiotics to the cement used for fixation of the implant, this is followed by a minimum of 6 weeks antibiotic therapy. Two studies comparing one-stage to two stage revision arthroplasty favoured the two stage technique[154, 155]. Failure rates in SSRA ranged from 10.1% to 12.4%, compared to 3.5% to 5.6% in TSRA. A recent meta-analysis comparing SSRA to TSRA reported the presence of nearly three additional reinfections per 100 revisions when performing a one stage compared to a two stage procedure[156]. However, not enough evidence is available to demonstrate that one technique is superior to the other[156].

5.5. Two stage revision arthroplasty

Two stage revision arthroplasty (TSRA) is currently the gold standard technique for the treatment of infected joint arthroplasty[107, 157-159]. TSRA involves initial removal of the infected components and all foreign material including cement, cement restrictors and cables or wires whenever possible with meticulous debridement and irrigation. All necrotic tissue is excised, and sinus tracts are debrided. After irrigation the joint should be inspected for any remaining debris. A cement spacer loaded with antibiotics is used, this is either pre-manufactured or constructed at the time of surgery[160, 161]. Various techniques described in the construction of a cement loaded spacer, the technique used depends on the joint involved and the level of bone loss encountered during the first stage[109, 161-164]. These custom spacers allow antibiotic elution locally to eradicate the infective organism and maintain soft tissue balance to accommodate the definitive implant during the second stage. A minimum course of six weeks of antibiotics is usually required, and resolution of infection is confirmed through serial ESR and CRP and repeated aspiration of the joint. A further aspiration of the joint before the second stage is recommended in one study, which reported recurrence rate of 3% among those who underwent aspiration compared with 14% in those who did not[165].

The advantages of TSRA[166] include:

i.   meticulous debridement of soft tissue, necrotic bone and cement during the first stage and during the second stage before reimplantation

ii.   identification of offending organism, sensitivities are determined and appropriate antibiotic therapy is given for a prolonged period before reimplantation

iii. evaluation of distant foci of infection and eradication of sites responsible for haematogenous spread

iv.   informed decision can be made as to whether the degree of disability from resection arthroplasty or arthrodesis would justify the risks involved in the implantation of a new prosthesis

The disadvantages[166] include:

i.   prolonged period of disability and hospital stay

ii.   increased costs

iii.   delayed rehabilitation

iv.   technically difficult second procedure due to loss soft tissue balance, loss of bone stock shortening and scarring

TSRA has been associated with lower rates of recurrent infections in most studies[6, 167, 168]. The duration of antibiotics between the two stages has not been determined, but a minimum of 6 weeks is usually standard and is guided by serial ESR and CRP levels. Management of bone stock deficiency at the time of revision is a problem. Impaction bone grafting with cemented prosthesis has been used for reconstruction during the second stage with good results. English et al. reported eradication in 49 out of 53 cases treated with impaction bone grafting during the second stage with a minimum follow up of 2 years[169] and a recurrence rate up to 7.5%[169, 170]. Use of antibiotic loaded cement for fixation of the implant during the second stage has been shown to reduce rates of reinfection. Garvin et al. reported eradication in 95% of patients at 5 year interval when gentamicin loaded cement was utilised during the second stage[171]. Highest success rates for TSRA were found for patients treated with antibiotics-eluting spacer or beads between the first and second stage, followed by a second reconstruction with an antibiotic loaded cemented reconstruction[55, 167, 172].

Data on uncemented implants has generally been less positive, with early studies reporting rates of infection as high as 18% and additional cases of loosening[43, 173]. Studies that are more recent have reported reinfection rates between 6% and 11%[174]. The decision regarding cemented or uncemented reimplantation is guided by the available bone stock, physiological age and expected longevity of the patient. To minimize loss of bone stock during the first stage, the Exeter group adopted a cement in cement revision technique for hip arthroplasty, where an excision arthroplasty with antibiotic impregnated cement beads is carried out during the first stage. In this technique if the cement mantle from the previous arthroplasty is well fixed, is left alone. During the second stage, the cement beads are removed, and the existing cement mantle is reamed to remove any membrane or microfilm and to create space for the new antibiotic augmented cement and the new implant. Sixteen patients with at least three years follow up underwent this procedure with one patient requiring revision due to recurrent infection[175].

5.6. Arthrodesis and amputation

Salvage procedures are reserved for patients whose medical condition such as immunocompromised patients or in patients where successful reconstruction is impossible. Successful reconstruction is limited those patients with insufficient bone stock, inadequate muscle function and poor soft tissue coverage. Eradication of infection after salvage procedures is reported between 86% to 96% although they are usually associated with poor functional outcomes[176-178]. Above knee amputation provides good return to function with a fitted prosthesis, especially in patients who cannot tolerate multiple procedures. Arthrodesis allows the patient to retain the extremity at the cost of reducing ambulation especially in patients with a fused knee.

6. Conclusion

Infection of a total Joint arthroplasty is considered a major complication in orthopaedic surgery with significant morbidity and places a considerable burden on hospitals and surgeons. Prevention is better than treatment and improving the patients' health prior to surgery is important in reducing the risk of infection. Furthermore, prompt diagnosis, permits early treatment that is important in acute infections. In the absence of a perfect test, the evidence based algorithmic approach brought forward by the AAOS guidelines should enable diagnosis of infection to be made with a high degree of confidence. There is clearly a role for surgical intervention, and so far a two-stage revision arthroplasty demonstrates the lowest rates of recurrent infection and as such is regarded as the 'gold standard'.

Author details

Adrian J. Cassar Gheiti and Kevin J. Mulhall

Orthopaedic Research and Innovation Foundation, Republic of Ireland

References

[1] Bozic KJ, Kurtz SM, Lau E, Ong K, Chiu V, Vail TP, et al. The epidemiology of revision total knee arthroplasty in the United States. Clin Orthop Relat Res. 2010;468[1]: 45-51. Epub 2009/06/26.

[2] Bozic KJ, Kurtz SM, Lau E, Ong K, Vail TP, Berry DJ. The epidemiology of revision total hip arthroplasty in the United States. J Bone Joint Surg Am. 2009;91[1]:128-33. Epub 2009/01/06.

[3] Clohisy JC, Calvert G, Tull F, McDonald D, Maloney WJ. Reasons for revision hip surgery: a retrospective review. Clin Orthop Relat Res. 2004[429]:188-92. Epub 2004/12/04.

[4] Vessely MB, Whaley AL, Harmsen WS, Schleck CD, Berry DJ. The Chitranjan Ranawat Award: Long-term survivorship and failure modes of 1000 cemented condylar total knee arthroplasties. Clin Orthop Relat Res. 2006;452:28-34. Epub 2006/08/29.

[5] Della Valle C, Parvizi J, Bauer TW, Dicesare PE, Evans RP, Segreti J, et al. Diagnosis of periprosthetic joint infections of the hip and knee. J Am Acad Orthop Surg. 2010;18[12]:760-70. Epub 2010/12/02.

[6] Parvizi J, Adeli B, Zmistowski B, Restrepo C, Greenwald AS. Management of Periprosthetic Joint Infection: The Current Knowledge: AAOS Exhibit Selection. J Bone Joint Surg Am. 2012;94[14]:e1041-9. Epub 2012/07/20.

[7] Parvizi J, Zmistowski B, Adeli B. Periprosthetic joint infection: treatment options. Orthopedics. 2010;33[9]:659. Epub 2010/09/16.

[8] Kurtz SM, Lau E, Watson H, Schmier JK, Parvizi J. Economic Burden of Periprosthetic Joint Infection in the United States. J Arthroplasty. 2012. Epub 2012/05/05.

[9] Bozic KJ, Lau E, Kurtz S, Ong K, Rubash H, Vail TP, et al. Patient-related risk factors for periprosthetic joint infection and postoperative mortality following total hip arthroplasty in Medicare patients. J Bone Joint Surg Am. 2012;94[9]:794-800. Epub 2012/05/04.

[10] Wilson MG, Kelley K, Thornhill TS. Infection as a complication of total knee-replacement arthroplasty. Risk factors and treatment in sixty-seven cases. J Bone Joint Surg Am. 1990;72[6]:878-83. Epub 1990/07/01.

[11] Zimmerli W, Trampuz A, Ochsner PE. Prosthetic-joint infections. N Engl J Med. 2004;351[16]:1645-54. Epub 2004/10/16.

[12] Pulido L, Ghanem E, Joshi A, Purtill JJ, Parvizi J. Periprosthetic joint infection: the incidence, timing, and predisposing factors. Clin Orthop Relat Res. 2008;466[7]:1710-5. Epub 2008/04/19.

[13] Sendi P, Banderet F, Graber P, Zimmerli W. Clinical comparison between exogenous and haematogenous periprosthetic joint infections caused by Staphylococcus aureus. Clin Microbiol Infect. 2011;17[7]:1098-100. Epub 2011/05/21.

[14] Greenky M, Gandhi K, Pulido L, Restrepo C, Parvizi J. Preoperative Anemia in Total Joint Arthroplasty: Is It Associated with Periprosthetic Joint Infection? Clin Orthop Relat Res. 2012. Epub 2012/07/10.

[15] Jafari SM, Casper DS, Restrepo C, Zmistowski B, Parvizi J, Sharkey PF. Periprosthetic joint infection: are patients with multiple prosthetic joints at risk? J Arthroplasty. 2012;27[6]:877-80. Epub 2012/03/06.

[16] Katthagen BD, Zamani P, Jung W. [Effect of surgical draping on bacterial contamination in the surgical field]. Z Orthop Ihre Grenzgeb. 1992;130[3]:230-5. Epub 1992/05/01. Einfluss der Inzisionsfolie auf das Keimverhalten im Operationsgebiet.

[17] Evans RP. Current concepts for clean air and total joint arthroplasty: laminar airflow and ultraviolet radiation: a systematic review. Clin Orthop Relat Res. 2011;469[4]: 945-53. Epub 2010/12/17.

[18] Panahi P, Stroh M, Casper DS, Parvizi J, Austin MS. Operating Room Traffic is a Major Concern During Total Joint Arthroplasty. Clin Orthop Relat Res. 2012. Epub 2012/02/04.

[19] Kearns KA, Witmer D, Makda J, Parvizi J, Jungkind D. Sterility of the personal protection system in total joint arthroplasty. Clin Orthop Relat Res. 2011;469[11]:3065-9. Epub 2011/06/15.

[20] Buller LT, Sabry FY, Easton RW, Klika AK, Barsoum WK. The preoperative prediction of success following irrigation and debridement with polyethylene exchange for hip and knee prosthetic joint infections. J Arthroplasty. 2012;27[6]:857-64 e1-4. Epub 2012/03/10.

[21] Jamsen E, Huhtala H, Puolakka T, Moilanen T. Risk factors for infection after knee arthroplasty. A register-based analysis of 43,149 cases. J Bone Joint Surg Am. 2009;91[1]:38-47. Epub 2009/01/06.

[22] Berbari EF, Hanssen AD, Duffy MC, Steckelberg JM, Ilstrup DM, Harmsen WS, et al. Risk factors for prosthetic joint infection: case-control study. Clin Infect Dis. 1998;27[5]:1247-54. Epub 1998/11/25.

[23] Saleh K, Olson M, Resig S, Bershadsky B, Kuskowski M, Gioe T, et al. Predictors of wound infection in hip and knee joint replacement: results from a 20 year surveillance program. J Orthop Res. 2002;20[3]:506-15. Epub 2002/06/01.

[24] Jamsen E, Nevalainen P, Eskelinen A, Huotari K, Kalliovalkama J, Moilanen T. Obesity, diabetes, and preoperative hyperglycemia as predictors of periprosthetic joint infection: a single-center analysis of 7181 primary hip and knee replacements for osteoarthritis. J Bone Joint Surg Am. 2012;94[14]:e1011-9. Epub 2012/07/20.

[25] Poss R, Thornhill TS, Ewald FC, Thomas WH, Batte NJ, Sledge CB. Factors influencing the incidence and outcome of infection following total joint arthroplasty. Clin Orthop Relat Res. 1984[182]:117-26. Epub 1984/01/01.

[26] Muilwijk J, van den Hof S, Wille JC. Associations between surgical site infection risk and hospital operation volume and surgeon operation volume among hospitals in the Dutch nosocomial infection surveillance network. Infect Control Hosp Epidemiol. 2007;28[5]:557-63. Epub 2007/04/28.

[27] Ong KL, Lau E, Manley M, Kurtz SM. Effect of procedure duration on total hip arthroplasty and total knee arthroplasty survivorship in the United States Medicare population. J Arthroplasty. 2008;23[6 Suppl 1]:127-32. Epub 2008/06/17.

[28] Fogelberg EV, Zitzmann EK, Stinchfield FE. Prophylactic penicillin in orthopaedic surgery. J Bone Joint Surg Am. 1970;52[1]:95-8. Epub 1970/01/01.

[29] Pavel A, Smith RL, Ballard A, Larsen IJ. Prophylactic antibiotics in clean orthopaedic surgery. J Bone Joint Surg Am. 1974;56[4]:777-82. Epub 1974/06/01.

[30] Meehan J, Jamali AA, Nguyen H. Prophylactic antibiotics in hip and knee arthroplasty. J Bone Joint Surg Am. 2009;91[10]:2480-90. Epub 2009/10/03.

[31] Al-Maiyah M, Hill D, Bajwa A, Slater S, Patil P, Port A, et al. Bacterial contaminants and antibiotic prophylaxis in total hip arthroplasty. J Bone Joint Surg Br. 2005;87[9]: 1256-8. Epub 2005/09/01.

[32] Hanssen AD. Prophylactic use of antibiotic bone cement: an emerging standard--in opposition. J Arthroplasty. 2004;19[4 Suppl 1]:73-7. Epub 2004/06/11.

[33] Johnson AJ, Daley JA, Zywiel MG, Delanois RE, Mont MA. Preoperative chlorhexidine preparation and the incidence of surgical site infections after hip arthroplasty. J Arthroplasty. 2010;25[6 Suppl):98-102. Epub 2010/06/24.

[34] Ayers DC DD, Johanson NA, Pellegrini.VD Jr. Instructional Course Lectures, The American Academy of Orthopaedic Surgeons - Common Complications of Total Knee Arthroplasty. J Bone Joint Surg Am. 1997;79[2]:278-311.

[35] Rao N, Cannella B, Crossett LS, Yates AJ, Jr., McGough R, 3rd. A preoperative decolonization protocol for staphylococcus aureus prevents orthopaedic infections. Clin Orthop Relat Res. 2008;466[6]:1343-8. Epub 2008/04/12.

[36] Gristina AG. Biomaterial-centered infection: microbial adhesion versus tissue integration. Science. 1987;237[4822]:1588-95. Epub 1987/09/25.

[37] Costerton JW, Stewart PS, Greenberg EP. Bacterial biofilms: a common cause of persistent infections. Science. 1999;284[5418]:1318-22. Epub 1999/05/21.

[38] Anderl JN, Zahller J, Roe F, Stewart PS. Role of nutrient limitation and stationary-phase existence in Klebsiella pneumoniae biofilm resistance to ampicillin and ciprofloxacin. Antimicrob Agents Chemother. 2003;47[4]:1251-6. Epub 2003/03/26.

[39] Darouiche RO. Device-associated infections: a macroproblem that starts with microadherence. Clin Infect Dis. 2001;33[9]:1567-72. Epub 2001/09/29.

[40] Hoiby N, Ciofu O, Johansen HK, Song ZJ, Moser C, Jensen PO, et al. The clinical impact of bacterial biofilms. International journal of oral science. 2011;3[2]:55-65. Epub 2011/04/13.

[41] Zimmerli W, Lew PD, Waldvogel FA. Pathogenesis of foreign body infection. Evidence for a local granulocyte defect. J Clin Invest. 1984;73[4]:1191-200. Epub 1984/04/01.

[42] Murdoch DR, Roberts SA, Fowler Jr VG, Jr., Shah MA, Taylor SL, Morris AJ, et al. Infection of orthopedic prostheses after Staphylococcus aureus bacteremia. Clin Infect Dis. 2001;32[4]:647-9. Epub 2001/02/22.

[43] Salvati EA, Gonzalez Della Valle A, Masri BA, Duncan CP. The infected total hip arthroplasty. Instr Course Lect. 2003;52:223-45. Epub 2003/04/15.

[44] Phillips JE, Crane TP, Noy M, Elliott TS, Grimer RJ. The incidence of deep prosthetic infections in a specialist orthopaedic hospital: a 15-year prospective survey. J Bone Joint Surg Br. 2006;88[7]:943-8. Epub 2006/06/27.

[45] Romano CL, Romano D, Logoluso N, Meani E. Septic versus aseptic hip revision: how different? J Orthop Traumatol. 2010;11[3]:167-74. Epub 2010/09/03.

[46] Zmistowski B, Fedorka CJ, Sheehan E, Deirmengian G, Austin MS, Parvizi J. Prosthetic joint infection caused by gram-negative organisms. J Arthroplasty. 2011;26[6 Suppl):104-8. Epub 2011/06/07.

[47] Anagnostakos K, Kelm J, Schmitt E, Jung J. Fungal periprosthetic hip and knee joint infections clinical experience with a 2-stage treatment protocol. J Arthroplasty. 2012;27[2]:293-8. Epub 2011/07/15.

[48] Mahmud T, Lyons MC, Naudie DD, Macdonald SJ, McCalden RW. Assessing the Gold Standard: A Review of 253 Two-Stage Revisions for Infected TKA. Clin Orthop Relat Res. 2012. Epub 2012/04/28.

[49] Hare R, Thomas CG. The transmission of Staphylococcus aureus. Br Med J. 1956;2[4997]:840-4. Epub 1956/10/13.

[50] Ritter MA. Operating room environment. Clin Orthop Relat Res. 1999[369]:103-9. Epub 1999/12/28.

[51] Passaro DJ, Waring L, Armstrong R, Bolding F, Bouvier B, Rosenberg J, et al. Postoperative Serratia marcescens wound infections traced to an out-of-hospital source. J Infect Dis. 1997;175[4]:992-5. Epub 1997/04/01.

[52] Veber B, Gachot B, Bedos JP, Wolff M. Severe sepsis after intravenous injection of contaminated propofol. Anesthesiology. 1994;80[3]:712-3. Epub 1994/03/01.

[53] Elek SD, Conen PE. The virulence of Staphylococcus pyogenes for man; a study of the problems of wound infection. Br J Exp Pathol. 1957;38[6]:573-86. Epub 1957/12/01.

[54] Zimmerli W, Waldvogel FA, Vaudaux P, Nydegger UE. Pathogenesis of foreign body infection: description and characteristics of an animal model. J Infect Dis. 1982;146[4]:487-97. Epub 1982/10/01.

[55] Fitzgerald RH, Jr., Nolan DR, Ilstrup DM, Van Scoy RE, Washington JA, 2nd, Coventry MB. Deep wound sepsis following total hip arthroplasty. J Bone Joint Surg Am. 1977;59[7]:847-55. Epub 1977/10/01.

[56] Tsukayama DT, Estrada R, Gustilo RB. Infection after total hip arthroplasty. A study of the treatment of one hundred and six infections. J Bone Joint Surg Am. 1996;78[4]:512-23. Epub 1996/04/01.

[57] Zimmerli W, Moser C. Pathogenesis and treatment concepts of orthopaedic biofilm infections. FEMS Immunol Med Microbiol. 2012;65[2]:158-68. Epub 2012/02/09.

[58] Maderazo EG, Judson S, Pasternak H. Late infections of total joint prostheses. A re-view and recommendations for prevention. Clin Orthop Relat Res. 1988[229]:131-42. Epub 1988/04/01.

[59] Workgroup Convened by the Musculoskeletal Infection S. New definition for peri-prosthetic joint infection. J Arthroplasty. 2011;26[8]:1136-8. Epub 2011/11/15.

[60] Malinzak RA, Ritter MA, Berend ME, Meding JB, Olberding EM, Davis KE. Morbidly obese, diabetic, younger, and unilateral joint arthroplasty patients have elevated total joint arthroplasty infection rates. J Arthroplasty. 2009;24[6 Suppl):84-8. Epub 2009/07/17.

[61] Fletcher N, Sofianos D, Berkes MB, Obremskey WT. Prevention of perioperative in-fection. J Bone Joint Surg Am. 2007;89[7]:1605-18. Epub 2007/07/04.

[62] Lai K, Bohm ER, Burnell C, Hedden DR. Presence of medical comorbidities in pa-tients with infected primary hip or knee arthroplasties. J Arthroplasty. 2007;22[5]: 651-6. Epub 2007/08/11.

[63] Kamal T, Conway RM, Littlejohn I, Ricketts D. The role of a multidisciplinary pre-assessment clinic in reducing mortality after complex orthopaedic surgery. Ann R Coll Surg Engl. 2011;93[2]:149-51. Epub 2011/11/02.

[64] Control CfD. Guidline For Prevention of Surgical Site Infection. 1999; Available from: http://www.cdc.gov/HAI/ssi/ssi.html.

[65] Bleasdale SC, Trick WE, Gonzalez IM, Lyles RD, Hayden MK, Weinstein RA. Effec-tiveness of chlorhexidine bathing to reduce catheter-associated bloodstream infec-tions in medical intensive care unit patients. Arch Intern Med. 2007;167[19]:2073-9. Epub 2007/10/24.

[66] Climo MW, Sepkowitz KA, Zuccotti G, Fraser VJ, Warren DK, Perl TM, et al. The ef-fect of daily bathing with chlorhexidine on the acquisition of methicillin-resistant Staphylococcus aureus, vancomycin-resistant Enterococcus, and healthcare-associat-ed bloodstream infections: results of a quasi-experimental multicenter trial. Crit Care Med. 2009;37[6]:1858-65. Epub 2009/04/23.

[67] Rao N, Cannella BA, Crossett LS, Yates AJ, Jr., McGough RL, 3rd, Hamilton CW. Pre-operative screening/decolonization for Staphylococcus aureus to prevent orthopedic surgical site infection: prospective cohort study with 2-year follow-up. J Arthroplas-ty. 2011;26[8]:1501-7. Epub 2011/04/22.

[68] Edmiston CE, Jr., Seabrook GR, Johnson CP, Paulson DS, Beausoleil CM. Compara-tive of a new and innovative 2% chlorhexidine gluconate-impregnated cloth with 4% chlorhexidine gluconate as topical antiseptic for preparation of the skin prior to sur-gery. Am J Infect Control. 2007;35[2]:89-96. Epub 2007/03/01.

[69] Ramos N, Skeete F, Haas JP, Hutzler L, Slover J, Phillips M, et al. Surgical site infec-tion prevention initiative - patient attitude and compliance. Bull NYU Hosp Jt Dis. 2011;69[4]:312-5. Epub 2011/12/27.

[70] Zywiel MG, Daley JA, Delanois RE, Naziri Q, Johnson AJ, Mont MA. Advance pre-operative chlorhexidine reduces the incidence of surgical site infections in knee arthroplasty. Int Orthop. 2011;35[7]:1001-6. Epub 2010/06/22.

[71] Eiselt D. Presurgical skin preparation with a novel 2% chlorhexidine gluconate cloth reduces rates of surgical site infection in orthopaedic surgical patients. Orthop Nurs. 2009;28[3]:141-5. Epub 2009/06/06.

[72] Mauerhan DR, Nelson CL, Smith DL, Fitzgerald RH, Jr., Slama TG, Petty RW, et al. Prophylaxis against infection in total joint arthroplasty. One day of cefuroxime compared with three days of cefazolin. J Bone Joint Surg Am. 1994;76[1]:39-45. Epub 1994/01/01.

[73] Tanner J, Norrie P, Melen K. Preoperative hair removal to reduce surgical site infection. Cochrane Database Syst Rev. 2011[11]:CD004122. Epub 2011/11/11.

[74] Edwards PS, Lipp A, Holmes A. Preoperative skin antiseptics for preventing surgical wound infections after clean surgery. Cochrane Database Syst Rev. 2004[3]:CD003949. Epub 2004/07/22.

[75] Ostrander RV, Brage ME, Botte MJ. Bacterial skin contamination after surgical preparation in foot and ankle surgery. Clin Orthop Relat Res. 2003[406]:246-52. Epub 2003/02/13.

[76] Keblish DJ, Zurakowski D, Wilson MG, Chiodo CP. Preoperative skin preparation of the foot and ankle: bristles and alcohol are better. J Bone Joint Surg Am. 2005;87[5]: 986-92. Epub 2005/05/04.

[77] Ostrander RV, Botte MJ, Brage ME. Efficacy of surgical preparation solutions in foot and ankle surgery. J Bone Joint Surg Am. 2005;87[5]:980-5. Epub 2005/05/04.

[78] Tanner J, Swarbrook S, Stuart J. Surgical hand antisepsis to reduce surgical site infection. Cochrane Database Syst Rev. 2008[1]:CD004288. Epub 2008/02/07.

[79] Larson EL, Butz AM, Gullette DL, Laughon BA. Alcohol for surgical scrubbing? Infect Control Hosp Epidemiol. 1990;11[3]:139-43. Epub 1990/03/01.

[80] French ML, Eitzen HE, Ritter MA. The plastic surgical adhesive drape: an evaluation of its efficacy as a microbial barrier. Ann Surg. 1976;184[1]:46-50. Epub 1976/07/01.

[81] Johnston DH, Fairclough JA, Brown EM, Morris R. Rate of bacterial recolonization of the skin after preparation: four methods compared. Br J Surg. 1987;74[1]:64. Epub 1987/01/01.

[82] Blom AW, Gozzard C, Heal J, Bowker K, Estela CM. Bacterial strike-through of re-usable surgical drapes: the effect of different wetting agents. J Hosp Infect. 2002;52[1]:52-5. Epub 2002/10/10.

[83] Blom A, Estela C, Bowker K, MacGowan A, Hardy JR. The passage of bacteria through surgical drapes. Ann R Coll Surg Engl. 2000;82[6]:405-7. Epub 2000/12/05.

[84]   Ritter MA, Campbell ED. Retrospective evaluation of an iodophor-incorporated anti-
       microbial plastic adhesive wound drape. Clin Orthop Relat Res. 1988[228]:307-8.
       Epub 1988/03/01.

[85]   Webster J, Alghamdi AA. Use of plastic adhesive drapes during surgery for prevent-
       ing surgical site infection. Cochrane Database Syst Rev. 2007[4]:CD006353. Epub
       2007/10/19.

[86]   Guo YP, Wong PM, Li Y, Or PP. Is double-gloving really protective? A comparison
       between the glove perforation rate among perioperative nurses with single and dou-
       ble gloves during surgery. Am J Surg. 2012;204[2]:210-5. Epub 2012/02/22.

[87]   Tanner J, Parkinson H. Double gloving to reduce surgical cross-infection. Cochrane
       Database Syst Rev. 2006[3]:CD003087. Epub 2006/07/21.

[88]   Ersozlu S, Sahin O, Ozgur AF, Akkaya T, Tuncay C. Glove punctures in major and
       minor orthopaedic surgery with double gloving. Acta Orthop Belg. 2007;73[6]:760-4.
       Epub 2008/02/12.

[89]   Beldame J, Lagrave B, Lievain L, Lefebvre B, Frebourg N, Dujardin F. Surgical glove
       bacterial contamination and perforation during total hip arthroplasty implantation:
       when gloves should be changed. Orthop Traumatol Surg Res. 2012;98[4]:432-40.
       Epub 2012/05/15.

[90]   Lidwell OM, Elson RA, Lowbury EJ, Whyte W, Blowers R, Stanley SJ, et al. Ultra-
       clean air and antibiotics for prevention of postoperative infection. A multicenter
       study of 8,052 joint replacement operations. Acta Orthop Scand. 1987;58[1]:4-13.
       Epub 1987/02/01.

[91]   Dharan S, Pittet D. Environmental controls in operating theatres. J Hosp Infect.
       2002;51[2]:79-84. Epub 2002/07/02.

[92]   Ayliffe GA. Role of the environment of the operating suite in surgical wound infec-
       tion. Rev Infect Dis. 1991;13 Suppl 10:S800-4. Epub 1991/09/01.

[93]   Gastmeier P, Breier AC, Brandt C. Influence of laminar airflow on prosthetic joint in-
       fections: a systematic review. J Hosp Infect. 2012;81[2]:73-8. Epub 2012/05/15.

[94]   Lynch RJ, Englesbe MJ, Sturm L, Bitar A, Budhiraj K, Kolla S, et al. Measurement of
       foot traffic in the operating room: implications for infection control. Am J Med Qual.
       2009;24[1]:45-52. Epub 2009/01/14.

[95]   Parikh SN, Grice SS, Schnell BM, Salisbury SR. Operating room traffic: is there any
       role of monitoring it? J Pediatr Orthop. 2010;30[6]:617-23. Epub 2010/08/25.

[96]   Charnley J, Eftekhar N. Penetration of gown material by organisms from the sur-
       geon's body. Lancet. 1969;1[7587]:172-3. Epub 1969/01/25.

[97]   Der Tavitian J, Ong SM, Taub NA, Taylor GJ. Body-exhaust suit versus occlusive
       clothing. A randomised, prospective trial using air and wound bacterial counts. J
       Bone Joint Surg Br. 2003;85[4]:490-4. Epub 2003/06/10.

[98] Howard JL, Hanssen AD. Principles of a clean operating room environment. J Arthroplasty. 2007;22[7 Suppl 3]:6-11. Epub 2007/11/21.

[99] Pasquarella C, Pitzurra O, Herren T, Poletti L, Savino A. Lack of influence of body exhaust gowns on aerobic bacterial surface counts in a mixed-ventilation operating theatre. A study of 62 hip arthroplasties. J Hosp Infect. 2003;54[1]:2-9. Epub 2003/05/28.

[100] Sanzen L, Carlsson AS, Walder M. Air contamination during total hip arthroplasty in an ultraclean air enclosure using different types of staff clothing. J Arthroplasty. 1990;5[2]:127-30. Epub 1990/06/01.

[101] Shaw JA, Bordner MA, Hamory BH. Efficacy of the Steri-Shield filtered exhaust helmet in limiting bacterial counts in the operating room during total joint arthroplasty. J Arthroplasty. 1996;11[4]:469-73. Epub 1996/06/01.

[102] Urquhart DM, Hanna FS, Brennan SL, Wluka AE, Leder K, Cameron PA, et al. Incidence and risk factors for deep surgical site infection after primary total hip arthroplasty: a systematic review. J Arthroplasty. 2010;25[8]:1216-22 e1-3. Epub 2009/11/03.

[103] Ong KL, Kurtz SM, Lau E, Bozic KJ, Berry DJ, Parvizi J. Prosthetic joint infection risk after total hip arthroplasty in the Medicare population. J Arthroplasty. 2009;24[6 Suppl):105-9. Epub 2009/06/06.

[104] Peersman G, Laskin R, Davis J, Peterson M. Infection in total knee replacement: a retrospective review of 6489 total knee replacements. Clin Orthop Relat Res. 2001[392]: 15-23. Epub 2001/11/22.

[105] Kurtz SM, Ong KL, Lau E, Bozic KJ, Berry D, Parvizi J. Prosthetic joint infection risk after TKA in the Medicare population. Clin Orthop Relat Res. 2010;468[1]:52-6. Epub 2009/08/12.

[106] Engesaeter LB, Lie SA, Espehaug B, Furnes O, Vollset SE, Havelin LI. Antibiotic prophylaxis in total hip arthroplasty: effects of antibiotic prophylaxis systemically and in bone cement on the revision rate of 22,170 primary hip replacements followed 0-14 years in the Norwegian Arthroplasty Register. Acta Orthop Scand. 2003;74[6]:644-51. Epub 2004/02/07.

[107] Romano CL, Romano D, Logoluso N, Meani E. Long-stem versus short-stem preformed antibiotic-loaded cement spacers for two-stage revision of infected total hip arthroplasty. Hip Int. 2010;20[1]:26-33. Epub 2010/03/18.

[108] Dairaku K, Takagi M, Kawaji H, Sasaki K, Ishii M, Ogino T. Antibiotics-impregnated cement spacers in the first step of two-stage revision for infected totally replaced hip joints: report of ten trial cases. J Orthop Sci. 2009;14[6]:704-10. Epub 2009/12/10.

[109] Cassar Gheiti AJ, Baker JF, Brown TE, Mulhall KJ. Management of Total Femoral Bone Loss Using a Hybrid Cement Spacer Surgical Technique. J Arthroplasty. 2012. Epub 2012/07/04.

[110] Chiu FY, Lin CF, Chen CM, Lo WH, Chaung TY. Cefuroxime-impregnated cement at primary total knee arthroplasty in diabetes mellitus. A prospective, randomised study. J Bone Joint Surg Br. 2001;83[5]:691-5. Epub 2001/07/31.

[111] Hanssen AD, Spangehl MJ. Practical applications of antibiotic-loaded bone cement for treatment of infected joint replacements. Clin Orthop Relat Res. 2004[427]:79-85. Epub 2004/11/24.

[112] Smith TO, Sexton D, Mann C, Donell S. Sutures versus staples for skin closure in orthopaedic surgery: meta-analysis. BMJ. 2010;340:c1199. Epub 2010/03/18.

[113] Newman JT, Morgan SJ, Resende GV, Williams AE, Hammerberg EM, Dayton MR. Modality of wound closure after total knee replacement: are staples as safe as sutures? A retrospective study of 181 patients. Patient Saf Surg. 2011;5[1]:26. Epub 2011/10/21.

[114] Eggers MD, Fang L, Lionberger DR. A comparison of wound closure techniques for total knee arthroplasty. J Arthroplasty. 2011;26[8]:1251-8 e1-4. Epub 2011/05/03.

[115] Patel RM, Cayo M, Patel A, Albarillo M, Puri L. Wound complications in joint arthroplasty: comparing traditional and modern methods of skin closure. Orthopedics. 2012;35[5]:e641-6. Epub 2012/05/17.

[116] Stephens S, Politi J, Taylor BC. Evaluation of Primary Total Knee Arthroplasty Incision Closure with the Use of Continuous Bidirectional Barbed Suture. Surg Technol Int. 2011;XXI:199-203. Epub 2012/04/17.

[117] Eickmann T, Quane E. Total knee arthroplasty closure with barbed sutures. J Knee Surg. 2010;23[3]:163-7. Epub 2011/02/19.

[118] Clarke JV, Deakin AH, Dillon JM, Emmerson S, Kinninmonth AW. A prospective clinical audit of a new dressing design for lower limb arthroplasty wounds. J Wound Care. 2009;18[1]:5-8, 10-1. Epub 2009/01/10.

[119] Cosker T, Elsayed S, Gupta S, Mendonca AD, Tayton KJ. Choice of dressing has a major impact on blistering and healing outcomes in orthopaedic patients. J Wound Care. 2005;14[1]:27-9. Epub 2005/01/20.

[120] Cho CY, Lo JS. Dressing the part. Dermatol Clin. 1998;16[1]:25-47. Epub 1998/02/14.

[121] Mertz PM, Marshall DA, Eaglstein WH. Occlusive wound dressings to prevent bacterial invasion and wound infection. J Am Acad Dermatol. 1985;12[4]:662-8. Epub 1985/04/01.

[122] Dumville JC, Walter CJ, Sharp CA, Page T. Dressings for the prevention of surgical site infection. Cochrane Database Syst Rev. 2011[7]:CD003091. Epub 2011/07/08.

[123] Burke NG, Green C, McHugh G, McGolderick N, Kilcoyne C, Kenny P. A prospective randomised study comparing the jubilee dressing method to a standard adhesive dressing for total hip and knee replacements. J Tissue Viability. 2012;21[3]:84-7. Epub 2012/06/05.

[124] Matar WY, Jafari SM, Restrepo C, Austin M, Purtill JJ, Parvizi J. Preventing infection in total joint arthroplasty. J Bone Joint Surg Am. 2010;92 Suppl 2:36-46. Epub 2010/12/09.

[125] Greidanus NV, Masri BA, Garbuz DS, Wilson SD, McAlinden MG, Xu M, et al. Use of erythrocyte sedimentation rate and C-reactive protein level to diagnose infection before revision total knee arthroplasty. A prospective evaluation. J Bone Joint Surg Am. 2007;89[7]:1409-16. Epub 2007/07/04.

[126] Schinsky MF, Della Valle CJ, Sporer SM, Paprosky WG. Perioperative testing for joint infection in patients undergoing revision total hip arthroplasty. J Bone Joint Surg Am. 2008;90[9]:1869-75. Epub 2008/09/03.

[127] Ghanem E, Antoci V, Jr., Pulido L, Joshi A, Hozack W, Parvizi J. The use of receiver operating characteristics analysis in determining erythrocyte sedimentation rate and C-reactive protein levels in diagnosing periprosthetic infection prior to revision total hip arthroplasty. Int J Infect Dis. 2009;13[6]:e444-9. Epub 2009/05/29.

[128] Toossi N, Adeli B, Rasouli MR, Huang R, Parvizi J. Serum White Blood Cell Count and Differential Do Not Have a Role in the Diagnosis of Periprosthetic Joint Infection. J Arthroplasty. 2012. Epub 2012/05/23.

[129] Trampuz A, Hanssen AD, Osmon DR, Mandrekar J, Steckelberg JM, Patel R. Synovial fluid leukocyte count and differential for the diagnosis of prosthetic knee infection. Am J Med. 2004;117[8]:556-62. Epub 2004/10/07.

[130] Ghanem E, Parvizi J, Burnett RS, Sharkey PF, Keshavarzi N, Aggarwal A, et al. Cell count and differential of aspirated fluid in the diagnosis of infection at the site of total knee arthroplasty. J Bone Joint Surg Am. 2008;90[8]:1637-43. Epub 2008/08/05.

[131] Tigges S, Stiles RG, Roberson JR. Appearance of septic hip prostheses on plain radiographs. AJR Am J Roentgenol. 1994;163[2]:377-80. Epub 1994/08/01.

[132] Smith SL, Wastie ML, Forster I. Radionuclide bone scintigraphy in the detection of significant complications after total knee joint replacement. Clin Radiol. 2001;56[3]: 221-4. Epub 2001/03/15.

[133] Love C, Marwin SE, Palestro CJ. Nuclear medicine and the infected joint replacement. Semin Nucl Med. 2009;39[1]:66-78. Epub 2008/11/29.

[134] Pandey R, Berendt AR, Athanasou NA. Histological and microbiological findings in non-infected and infected revision arthroplasty tissues. The OSIRIS Collaborative Study Group. Oxford Skeletal Infection Research and Intervention Service. Arch Orthop Trauma Surg. 2000;120[10]:570-4. Epub 2000/12/08.

[135] Atkins BL, Athanasou N, Deeks JJ, Crook DW, Simpson H, Peto TE, et al. Prospective evaluation of criteria for microbiological diagnosis of prosthetic-joint infection at revision arthroplasty. The OSIRIS Collaborative Study Group. J Clin Microbiol. 1998;36[10]:2932-9. Epub 1998/09/17.

[136] Spangehl MJ, Masri BA, O'Connell JX, Duncan CP. Prospective analysis of preoperative and intraoperative investigations for the diagnosis of infection at the sites of two hundred and two revision total hip arthroplasties. J Bone Joint Surg Am. 1999;81[5]: 672-83. Epub 1999/06/09.

[137] Johnson AJ, Zywiel MG, Stroh DA, Marker DR, Mont MA. Should gram stains have a role in diagnosing hip arthroplasty infections? Clin Orthop Relat Res. 2010;468[9]: 2387-91. Epub 2010/01/06.

[138] Oethinger M, Warner DK, Schindler SA, Kobayashi H, Bauer TW. Diagnosing periprosthetic infection: false-positive intraoperative Gram stains. Clin Orthop Relat Res. 2011;469[4]:954-60. Epub 2010/10/01.

[139] Parvizi J, Jacovides C, Antoci V, Ghanem E. Diagnosis of periprosthetic joint infection: the utility of a simple yet unappreciated enzyme. J Bone Joint Surg Am. 2011;93[24]:2242-8. Epub 2012/01/20.

[140] Wetters NG, Berend KR, Lombardi AV, Morris MJ, Tucker TL, Della Valle CJ. Leukocyte Esterase Reagent Strips for the Rapid Diagnosis of Periprosthetic Joint Infection. J Arthroplasty. 2012. Epub 2012/05/23.

[141] Parvizi J, Jacovides C, Adeli B, Jung KA, Hozack WJ. Mark B. Coventry Award: synovial C-reactive protein: a prospective evaluation of a molecular marker for periprosthetic knee joint infection. Clin Orthop Relat Res. 2012;470[1]:54-60. Epub 2011/07/26.

[142] Parvizi J, McKenzie JC, Cashman JP. Diagnosis of Periprosthetic Joint Infection Using Synovial C-Reactive Protein. J Arthroplasty. 2012. Epub 2012/05/09.

[143] Jacovides CL, Parvizi J, Adeli B, Jung KA. Molecular markers for diagnosis of periprosthetic joint infection. J Arthroplasty. 2011;26[6 Suppl]:99-103 e1. Epub 2011/05/17.

[144] Della Valle C, Parvizi J., Bauer T.W., DiCesare, P.E., Evans, R.P., Segreti, J., Spangehl, M. Diagnosis of Periprosthetic Joint Infections of the Hip and Knee. 2010; Available from: http://www.aaos.org/research/guidelines/PJIguideline.asp.

[145] Dupont JA. Significance of operative cultures in total hip arthroplasty. Clin Orthop Relat Res. 1986[211]:122-7. Epub 1986/10/01.

[146] Toms AD, Davidson D, Masri BA, Duncan CP. The management of peri-prosthetic infection in total joint arthroplasty. J Bone Joint Surg Br. 2006;88[2]:149-55. Epub 2006/01/26.

[147] Rao N, Crossett LS, Sinha RK, Le Frock JL. Long-term suppression of infection in total joint arthroplasty. Clin Orthop Relat Res. 2003[414]:55-60. Epub 2003/09/11.

[148] Segreti J, Nelson JA, Trenholme GM. Prolonged suppressive antibiotic therapy for infected orthopedic prostheses. Clin Infect Dis. 1998;27[4]:711-3. Epub 1998/11/03.

[149] Goulet JA, Pellicci PM, Brause BD, Salvati EM. Prolonged suppression of infection in total hip arthroplasty. J Arthroplasty. 1988;3[2]:109-16. Epub 1988/01/01.

[150] Crockarell JR, Hanssen AD, Osmon DR, Morrey BF. Treatment of infection with de-bridement and retention of the components following hip arthroplasty. J Bone Joint Surg Am. 1998;80[9]:1306-13. Epub 1998/10/06.

[151] Odum SM, Fehring TK, Lombardi AV, Zmistowski BM, Brown NM, Luna JT, et al. Irrigation and debridement for periprosthetic infections: does the organism matter? J Arthroplasty. 2011;26[6 Suppl):114-8. Epub 2011/05/31.

[152] Baker JF, Vioreanu MH, Harty JA. Clostridium perfringens infection complicating periprosthetic fracture fixation about the hip: successful treatment with early aggres-sive debridement. Hip Int. 2012;22[1]:122-5. Epub 2012/02/22.

[153] Callaghan JJ, Katz RP, Johnston RC. One-stage revision surgery of the infected hip. A minimum 10-year followup study. Clin Orthop Relat Res. 1999[369]:139-43. Epub 1999/12/28.

[154] Elson RA. Exchange arthroplasty for infection. Perspectives from the United King-dom. Orthop Clin North Am. 1993;24[4]:761-7. Epub 1993/10/01.

[155] Garvin KL, Fitzgerald RH, Jr., Salvati EA, Brause BD, Nercessian OA, Wallrichs SL, et al. Reconstruction of the infected total hip and knee arthroplasty with gentamicin-impregnated Palacos bone cement. Instr Course Lect. 1993;42:293-302. Epub 1993/01/01.

[156] Lange J, Troelsen A, Thomsen RW, Soballe K. Chronic infections in hip arthroplas-ties: comparing risk of reinfection following one-stage and two-stage revision: a sys-tematic review and meta-analysis. Clin Epidemiol. 2012;4:57-73. Epub 2012/04/14.

[157] Younger AS, Duncan CP, Masri BA, McGraw RW. The outcome of two-stage arthro-plasty using a custom-made interval spacer to treat the infected hip. J Arthroplasty. 1997;12[6]:615-23. Epub 1997/11/05.

[158] Garvin KL, Backstein D, Pellegrini VD, Jr., Kim RH, Lewallen DG. Dealing with com-plications. J Bone Joint Surg Am. 2009;91 Suppl 5:18-21. Epub 2009/08/08.

[159] Pignatti G, Nitta S, Rani N, Dallari D, Sabbioni G, Stagni C, et al. Two stage hip revi-sion in periprosthetic infection: results of 41 cases. Open Orthop J. 2010;4:193-200. Epub 2010/08/20.

[160] Wan Z, Momaya A, Karim A, Incavo SJ, Mathis KB. Preformed Articulating Knee Spacers in 2-Stage Total Knee Revision Arthroplasty: Minimum 2-Year Follow-Up. J Arthroplasty. 2012. Epub 2012/03/20.

[161] Duncan CP, Beauchamp C. A temporary antibiotic-loaded joint replacement system for management of complex infections involving the hip. Orthop Clin North Am. 1993;24[4]:751-9. Epub 1993/10/01.

[162] Richards C, Bell CJ, Viswanathan S, English H, Crawford RW. Use of a cement-load-ed Kuntscher nail in first-stage revision hip arthroplasty for massive femoral bone

loss secondary to infection: a report of four cases. J Orthop Surg (Hong Kong). 2010;18[1]:107-9. Epub 2010/04/30.

[163] Yoo J, Lee S, Han C, Chang J. The modified static spacers using antibiotic-impregnated cement rod in two-stage revision for infected total knee arthroplasty. Clin Orthop Surg. 2011;3[3]:245-8. Epub 2011/09/13.

[164] Morgan M TA, Hubble M.J.W. Diagnosis and Management of Infection. In: Ling RSM, Princess Elizabeth Orthopaedic Hospital. Exeter Hip U, editors. The Exeter hip : 40 years of innovation in total hip arthroplasty. Exeter: Exeter Hip Publishing; 2010. p. 369 p.

[165] Mont MA, Waldman BJ, Hungerford DS. Evaluation of preoperative cultures before second-stage reimplantation of a total knee prosthesis complicated by infection. A comparison-group study. J Bone Joint Surg Am. 2000;82-A[11]:1552-7. Epub 2000/11/30.

[166] Canale ST, Beaty JH. Part III - Arthroplasty. Campbell's operative orthopaedics. 11th ed. St. Louis, Mo. ; London: Mosby Elsevier; 2008.

[167] Hanssen AD, Rand JA. Evaluation and treatment of infection at the site of a total hip or knee arthroplasty. Instr Course Lect. 1999;48:111-22. Epub 1999/03/31.

[168] Choi HR, Malchau H, Bedair H. Are Prosthetic Spacers Safe to Use in 2-Stage Treatment for Infected Total Knee Arthroplasty? J Arthroplasty. 2012. Epub 2012/04/17.

[169] English H, Timperley AJ, Dunlop D, Gie G. Impaction grafting of the femur in two-stage revision for infected total hip replacement. J Bone Joint Surg Br. 2002;84[5]: 700-5. Epub 2002/08/22.

[170] Alexeeff M, Mahomed N, Morsi E, Garbuz D, Gross A. Structural allograft in two-stage revisions for failed septic hip arthroplasty. J Bone Joint Surg Br. 1996;78[2]: 213-6. Epub 1996/03/01.

[171] Garvin KL, Evans BG, Salvati EA, Brause BD. Palacos gentamicin for the treatment of deep periprosthetic hip infections. Clin Orthop Relat Res. 1994[298]:97-105. Epub 1994/01/01.

[172] Hanssen AD, Spangehl MJ. Treatment of the infected hip replacement. Clin Orthop Relat Res. 2004[420]:63-71. Epub 2004/04/02.

[173] Nestor BJ, Hanssen AD, Ferrer-Gonzalez R, Fitzgerald RH, Jr. The use of porous prostheses in delayed reconstruction of total hip replacements that have failed because of infection. J Bone Joint Surg Am. 1994;76[3]:349-59. Epub 1994/03/01.

[174] Mitchell PA, Masri BA, Garbuz DS, Greidanus NV, Duncan CP. Cementless revision for infection following total hip arthroplasty. Instr Course Lect. 2003;52:323-30. Epub 2003/04/15.

[175] Hubble MJW, Whittaker, J.P., Blake, S.M., Briant-Evans, T. Cement In Cement revision. In: Ling RSM, Princess Elizabeth Orthopaedic Hospital. Exeter Hip U, editors.

The Exeter hip : 40 years of innovation in total hip arthroplasty. Exeter: Exeter Hip Publishing; 2010. p. 369 p.

[176] Bourne RB, Hunter GA, Rorabeck CH, Macnab JJ. A six-year follow-up of infected total hip replacements managed by Girdlestone's arthroplasty. J Bone Joint Surg Br. 1984;66[3]:340-3. Epub 1984/05/01.

[177] Castellanos J, Flores X, Llusa M, Chiriboga C, Navarro A. The Girdlestone pseudarthrosis in the treatment of infected hip replacements. Int Orthop. 1998;22[3]:178-81. Epub 1998/09/05.

[178] Conway JD, Mont MA, Bezwada HP. Arthrodesis of the knee. J Bone Joint Surg Am. 2004;86-A[4]:835-48. Epub 2004/04/08.

Chapter 7

Periprosthetic Infection Following Total Knee Arthroplasty

Michael Soudry, Arnan Greental,
Gabriel Nierenberg, Mazen Falah and
Nahum Rosenberg

Additional information is available at the end of the chapter

1. Introduction

One of the most devastating complications of prosthetic knee arthroplasty is a periprosthetic infection. This complication occurs in 1-2% of knee arthroplasties [1,2] and can exceed 4% in immunocompromised individuals [3] and 7% after revision surgery [4]. Prosthetic infection leads to loosening of the implant, [5,6]. In this circumstances revision surgery is required. Because of the diversity of the clinical presentation, i.e. early, intermediate or late infection [1], different surgical methods to treat infected knee prostheses were developed [5,6]. Several treatment methods became well accepted but others are still controversial. In the present review we intend to describe mainly the diagnostic tools for detection of infection and commonly used treatment methods in failed total knee arthroplasty due to infection, with special emphasis on the surgical techniques. Additionally we will describe some trends for the future improvement of the treatment modalities.

2. Pathology and microbiology

The main infecting pathogens, around 50%, of knee prostheses, are the different strains of *Staphylococci*, e.g. coagulase negative *Staphylococci* cause around 27% of knee prostheses infections and *Staphylococcus aureus* is responsible for 23% of infections, according to pooled data from nine different studies [7]. Most of the clinically significant infections are caused by biofilm producing microorganisms. The role of biofilms in pathogenesis of periprosthetic infection is the masking of the pathogens from bodily immune response and antibiotic access. Biofilm is a biological structure containing bacteria in a planktonic form imbedded in extracellular matrix made of different polysaccharide molecules, proteins and extracellular DNA (Figure 1). Biofilm generation goes through four consecutive steps: adherence of the pathogens to the surface of prosthesis, accumulation of the biofilm components, maturation of the biofilm and finally its detachment and spread of the microorganisms [8]. The ability of the microorganism to produce masking biofilm defines its virulence in prosthetic infection. Commensal bacteria, such as coagulase negative *Staphylococci* are more frequent in immediate and early prosthetic infections, when spread from the surgical wound edges and in late low grade infections. In late infections by hematogeous spread the *Staphylococcus aureus* is the most important causative factor [9].

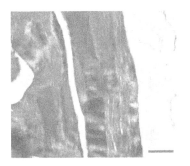

Figure 1. Microscopic image (H&E staining, scale 100µ) of biofilm found at the edge of retrieved tibial component of infected knee prosthesis. Amorphous fibrin-like substance, mostly acellular, is evident

3. Timing of occurence

Infections associated with prosthetic joints are classified according to time at detection as: early (develop less than 3 months after surgery), delayed [3 to 24 months after surgery) or late (more than 24 months after surgery) [10]. Clinical manifestations are in relation with timing [11]. In early cases clinical manifestations are joint pain, effusion, erythema and warmth of the joint. In delayed cases there are subtle signs such as implant loosening, persistent joint pain. Infection is generally provoked by less virulent microorganism. Late are acquired during hematogenous seeding. In a study of infection with THA during a 16 years period, 29 % of cases were early infections, 41 % delayed and 30% late infections [12].

4. Diagnosis

Accurate and early diagnosis is the first step in effectively managing patients with prosthetic joint infection. Clinical history, physical examination, laboratory data and imaging studies are all taken into consideration. In addition to cultures, the most commonly used laboratory tests include serum inflammatory markers and synovial fluid cytology.

Plain films: The appearance of rapidly progressive radiolucent lines surrounding an implant may be present during an infection. The resorption of subchondral bone and patchy osteoporosis are strong elements of suspicion (Figure 2).

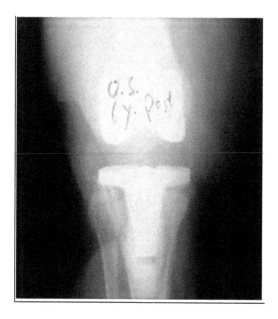

Figure 2. Radiograph of right knee (anterior-posterior view) showing radiolucency under the tibial component indicating periprosthetic infection.

Bone scan: bone scan can help confirm a diagnosis. However its high cost and its inability to provide acceptable levels of sensitivity and specificity have restricted its use. Although bone scintigraphy with technetium 99 m – labeled methylene diphosphonate has a high sensitivity, it lacks specificity for infection [13]. A technetium bone scan remains positive more than one year after implantation because of increased periprosthetic bone remodeling. Bone scan alone without labeling of the white cell has been found to have no role in diagnosing prosthetic joint infection. However, the use of indium 111 labeled leucocyte is time consuming and requires specialized labelling facility [14].

Laboratory tests: There is no evidence supporting the role of WBC and/or white cell blood differential in diagnosis of presence or absence of infection. ESR and CRP are valuable markers for both diagnosing and monitoring periprosthetic infection. After surgery the C Reactive protein level is elevated and return to normal within weeks. Serial postoperative measurements are more informative than single values [15].

Elevated serum interleukin-6 level correlated positively with the presence of periprosthetic infection in patients undergoing a reoperation at the site of a total hip or knee arthroplasty.

In a prospective, case-control study of 58 patients undergoing revision surgery of total hip and knee arthroplasties, serum Interleukin-6 values >10 pg/mL was reported to have a sensitivity of 100%, specificity of 95%, positive predictive value of 89%, negative predictive value of 100% and accuracy of 97% [16].

Knee aspirate cell count and differential: Synovial fluid cell count and differential is a very useful diagnostic test. Antibiotics should be suspended, if possible, for 10 to 14 days before carrying out the aspiration. Traumatic aspirations will result in falsely elevated leukocyte counts.

Polymerase chain reaction (PCR): This method is used to detect and amplify the presence of bacterial DNA. It is thought to be a quick method since it is not affected by whether the patient takes antibiotics or not. However, a high percentage of false negative test results has been detected [17]. Therefore currently this technique can be used as a complementary diagnostic tool to the methods described above.

Sonication: Organisms associated with prosthetic-joint infection are found attached to the prosthesis, where they often form biofilms. This suggests that obtaining a sample from the implant might improve the diagnosis of prosthetic joint infection by unmasking adherent bacteria from explanted prosthesis by sonication. It was found that culture of samples obtained by sonication of prostheses were more sensitive than conventional periprosthetic-tissue culture for the microbiologic diagnosis of prosthetic joint infection, especially in patients who had received antimicrobial therapy within 14 days before surgery [18].

Intraoperative Frozen Section: The analysis of frozen histological sections is a valuable tool for diagnosing infection. It most often used to assist decision-making in cases with equivocal serum inflammatory makers and aspirate cytology. The cutoff value of >5 neutrophils per high power field at a magnification of 400 is most commonly used for the diagnosis of infection. The sensitivity is more than 80 percent and a specificity of of more than 80 percent [19].

Intraoperative Gram Stain: This modality is unreliable (sensitivity = 27%) and should not be used routinely. The AAOS guideline recommends against the use of intraoperative gram stain to rule out periprosthetic infection [20].

5. Management of total knee arthroplasty infection

There are several options when it comes to managing an infected TKA. But before we select any of these, we must take into consideration a series of factors. These factors include the amount of time elapsed from infection, host-related factors, condition of the soft tissues, condition of the implant, virulence of microorganism present and its degree of sensitivity and, last but not least, the patient's expectations and functional needs.

Planning for any one option requires having detailed clinical records, cultures, x-rays and information of previously received treatment. It is important to identify high-risk patients, i.e. those receiving immunosuppressive treatment or suffering from malnutrition or systemic disease, trying to improve their general condition as much as possible before surgery.

Physical examination should provide information about the patient's neurovascular situation, articular mobility, the condition of their extensor mechanism and their soft tissues as well as about any previous incisions or the need of skin coverage by a plastic surgeon. Preoperative planning is important. The final goal of treatment is to eradicate infection, ease the pain and preserve the limb's function.

5.1. Antibiotic suppressive therapy

Efficiency of infection eradication with antibiotic therapy only is limited mainly due to the presence of foreign bodies, as implant and acrylic cement, and bacterial biofilm, therefore its use should be restricted to specific circumstances [21,22].

Indications for this type of treatment are as follows: 1) High operative risk due to medical co-morbidities; 2) Presence of low-virulence micro-organisms susceptible oral antibiotics that can be tolerated by the patient; 3) Mechanically stable prosthesis.

Antibiotic treatment should follow 3 basic principles: 1) Use of antibiotics of proven intracellular efficacy such as rifampicin, and new anti-staphylococcal agents. 2) Antibiotics should be combined, using a minimum of two to enhance the possibility of therapeutic success. 3) Long-standing administration, i.e. treatment should last a minimum of 6 months.

The use of new antibiotics could improve results for resistant bacteria. The oxazolidinone linezolid is a new wide-spectrum antibiotic with very attractive pharmacokinetic and activity profiles. It is an antibiotic that acts against methicillin-resistant staphylococci and vancomycin-resistant enterococci.

5.2. Surgical treatment

In early infection debridement and irrigation, without removing the implant, are usually chosen for surgical treatment.

The approach is through the previous surgical wound. Following division the subcutaneous tissue the knee is aspirated again.

Beforehand, the surgeon should carefully evaluate the knee radiographs for any sign of loosening, slight change in the components position, heterotrophic bone formation. All these may indicate chronic situation. Following the surgical exposure the stability of the implant should be evaluated. If reactive tissue found to sprout at the edge of the implant, it also might indicate on chronicity of the infection.[23, 24, 25]

Extensive debridement should be performed followed with vigorous irrigation. The debrided tissue is sent for cultures and pathology while the implant preserved. When no reactive tissue left, last survey should include the gutters, the patellar tracking and the back fold of the knee.

Closure of the knee might need multi layers sutures, using non absorbable materials over heavy drain, which could be left in place for several days to the discharge to stop. Most surgeons allow regular rehabilitation and long term IV antibiotics. Some surgeons leave antibiotic beads and perform recurrent debridement prior to knee rehabilitation [23]

5.3. Delayed or late infections

With delayed or late infection the orthopedic surgeon might face various clinical uncertainties with regard of decision making. The following are the most common clinical situations that are usually encountered:

Suppurating knee with positive cultures

Clinically infected knee with positive laboratory data but negative cultures

Clinically suspected infected knee without support of laboratory data

Clinically not infected knee with positive cultures

5.3.1. Suppurating knee with positive cultures

Identification of the infective germ prior to surgery allows preparation of appropriate antibiotics use within the operation. In some centers single stage revision preferred in cases of low virulence germ, effective antibiotics available both for embedding in the cement and the parenteral line.

Most surgeons favor a two-stage revision instead of a one-stage procedure [26, 27]

5.3.1.1. The two stage procedure

The two-stage procedure is indicated particularly to treat overt infections with an active discharge and virulent organism on culture such as *Staphylococus aureus* and mainly in methicillin-resistant staphylococcus (MRSA). Removal of the implant is done in first stage and implantation of the new prosthesis is performed later and delayed for a variable period of time until all parameters of inflammation disappear (Figure 3).

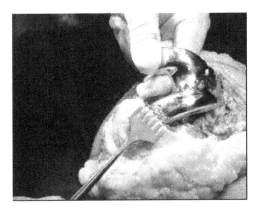

Figure 3. Intraoperative image of the grossly infected knee prosthesis before retrieval

The use of tourniquet without Esmarch bandage is advisable. Careful marking of the scars allows excision of the scars with old suture material. The arthrotomy should follow the original cut with extended lengths if necessary. Careful dissection is utilized in order to protect the vulnerable subcutaneous flaps. If open sinuses exist they should be debrided through the track. Pus and soft tissue are sent to culture with long incubation [28]. Extensive meticulous debridement is performed to the level of natural tissue, removing all synovial necrotic and non viable tissue. [27,29]. All prosthetic components and acrylic cement are removed.

After the implants are exposed from all soft tissue, the anterior surface of the femoral component is gently released as with Gigli saw, the distal part of it is detached by thin osteotome and gentle mallet percussions saving the bone stock, without leaning on the soft infected bone. Following removal of the femoral component the undersurface of the tibial tray is released with a saw and osteotomes which are inserted medially and laterally. Then hammering of the tray away from the tibia is performed. Meticulous removal of **all** pieces of cement **is a must** and,although can be technically demanding, should be accomplished. Thorough debridement is performed again with excision and removal of all remnants of infected tissue. Then the dressing is changed and the knee is draped again. Irrigation should follow with 3 to 4 liters of saline. Five minutes of betadine soaking of the wound should be followed by insertion of antibiotic-impregnated spacers.

A cement spacer impregnated with eluting antimicrobial drugs, according the sensitivity of the infective microorganism, is then interposed between distal femur and proximal tibia. This keeps the limb at its correct length and allows partial joint mobility Non-articulating, or articulated, spacers, can be used according to preference. Few spacer types are used: antibiotic cemented beads, antibiotic cement block, articulating spacer etc [30, 31, 32] (Figure 4).

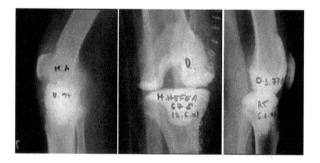

Figure 4. Knee radiographs showing different types of cement spacers

The non articulated spacer is a fixed one, with inherited stability that allows post op full weight bearing but no knee movement. Sometimes an intramedullary nail (abut 30-36 cm long) used to bridge the knee with cement for the enhanced stability. Care should be taken to prevent thermal injuries by the inserted cement at its' extension under the patella.

A divided or articulated spacer contains two parts: one piece should be attached to the proximal tibia and the other to the distal femur. The articulating cement spacer allows the patient to bend his knee, to exercise for range of movement, thus preventing joint contractures and keeping the extensor mechanism integrity.

Adequate hemostasis should follow tourniquet release, irrigation and closure of the wound over a large bore drain.

Antibiotics are administered intravenously according to microbial sensitivity for an average of six weeks. The interval can vary between the two stages, e.g. between six weeks to three months, when the clinical condition is settled. During this period, the clinical recovery is carefully evaluated by the laboratory tests for infection control (ESR and CRP). If there is no clear evidence of clinical improvement, re-arthrotomy and debridement should be considered.

The second stage requires re-arthrotomy through the old scar, tissue is sent for cultures, for pathologic examination, including high power field microscopic examination. The cement spacer is removed; the surgeon should patiently repeat the meticulous debridement. Intense irrigation and change of knee dressing followed by bone preparation and revision implant cementing are performed. A constrained rotating knee prosthesis is generally the most suitable implant particularly in cases of bone loss.

5.3.1.2. The one stage procedure

The use of a single-stage revision is advocated by some in certain patients with known causative organism, when no discharging sinuses are present, the patient is not immunocompromized, and there is no radiological evidence of component loosening or osteitis.

This type of revision is considered when pathogen germ has been definitely identified with appropriate sensitive antibiotic. The cement should contain suitable antibiotics according the sensitivity of the infective pathogen, if it is known; antimicrobial treatment is given 2-3 weeks before prosthesis exchange.

Technically one stage revision procedure includes removal of all foreign material, implant components and cement, thorough the same steps of meticulous debridement, as stated above, and re-implantation of a new prosthesis at the same surgical session.

5.3.2. Clinically infected knee with positive laboratory data but negative cultures

Clinical infection with negative cultures is not rare. A patient may present painful and swollen knee, with synovitis and intraarticular fluid, elevated ESR and CRP, with positive leukocyte bone scan, while aspirated fluid reveal negative cultures. In such a case the aspiration should be repeated, and microbiological studies for rare microorganisms, including PCR should be performed.

The clinical suspicion mandates the type of surgery: The surgical process should be identical to 1st stage revision with extensive debridement and removal of the implant. Multiple bone and soft tissue cultures and pathology should be obtained intraoperatively. Sonication of the prosthesis might be indicated. The cement spacer should contain antibiotics relevant against the common bacteria. Post operative intravenous antibiotics should be administered for six weeks. The 2nd stage is similar to those performed for the positive culture group.

The one-stage type of revision can also be considered in presence of low grade clinical expression, such as long relentless pain, local heat, tenderness and slow rehabilitation milestones, negative preoperative aspiration cultures and intraoperative gram stains, as well as frozen section demonstrating less than 5 polymorphonuclears per high power field. Aged patients with positive cultures for low virulence strains, such as *Staphylococcus epidermidis* and *Streptococcus type* A, are sometimes allocated for revision in a single stage.

5.3.3. Clinically suspected infected knee without support of laboratory data

This group of patients is presented with swollen painful knee, sometimes with synovitis and loosening. Usually not long from the primary surgery, with no sign of polyethylene wear, normal laboratory tests as CRP or ESR, normal blood leukocytes count and negative leukocytes bone scan. Knee aspiration could reveal not clear fluid but with negative culture. In such circumstances repeated aspiration performed and the workup should be extended for material allergy such as nickel and chrome. If the clinical suspicion for infection is significant the surgeon might take steps as for fully infected case, performing two or single stage revision. The decision making in these circumstances lacks a high level of evidence support.

5.3.4. Clinically not infected knee with positive cultures

Bone and soft tissue cultures are part of all knee revision as well as routine sonication of the retrieved implants. Sometimes a positive culture might be discovered in routine, not infected, with normal blood tests, negative leukocyte bone scan and without gross intraoperative signs of infected knee prosthesis. The finding should be carefully evaluated for contamination. If high suspicion for masked infection exists, six weeks of parenteral antibiotic should be administered.

6. Outcome of treatment with surgical revision

As a rule, revision Total Knee Arthroplasty offers inferior results and higher complication rates compared to primary arthroplasty [33].

According to the published data the successful functional results following the treatment of late infection of a total knee arthroplasty by a two-stage re-implantation of a new prosthesis should be expected in about 90% of patients [34, 35, 36, 37].

In spite of its high personal and financial burden the two-stage re-implantation is recognized as the most reliable method for eradicating infection [38]. Although one-stage revision is appealing and less technically demanding, the risk of re-infection is a deterring factor.

Two-stage revision procedures may encounter bone loss, obscure landmarks, structural weakness and soft tissue deficiency, which may result in continued pain, decreased mobility and rarely fractures. Nevertheless, the success rate of this method was found to be in the range of 82-93%, whereas the success rate of the one-stage procedure was of 71-81% [34]. Therefore two-stage re-implantation technique represents the procedure of choice for definitive eradication of infection and preservation of knee function.

According to the published data on one-stage revisions (Table 1) in the large series of patients, with mid-term follow up, around 80% success rate in eradication of infection should be expected.

Author	Year	No. of patients	Follow-up duration	Success rate*
Foerster et al[39]	1991	104	5-15 years	80%
Lu et al[49]	1997	8	20.1 months	100%
Siegel et al[50]	2000	31	2-15 years	71% (22/31)
Buechel et al[27]	2004	22	10.2 years	90.9%
Soudry et al[42]	2009	20	8 years	80% (16/20)

* Rates of infection eradication

Table 1. Results of one-stage knee revision arthroplasty

As early as 1983, Windsor and Insall reported a success rate of 97.4% in two-stage revision surgery in 38 patients, with four years of follow-up, but other reports had slightly lower success rates, around 90% (Table 2).

Author	Year	No. of patients	Average follow-up	Success rate*
Windsor & Insall [40]	1983	384	4 years	97.4%
Hannsen et al [51]	1994	36	52 months	89%
Goldman et al [52]	1996	64	7.5 years	97%
Gacon et al [53]	1997	29	3.5 years	82.7%
Hirakawa et al [53]	1998	55	61.9 months	87.2%
Siebel et al [55]	2002	10	13.5 months	100%
Pietsch et al [56]	2003	24	14.8 months	95.8%
Haleem et al [37]	2004	96	7.2 years	91%
Soudry et al [42]	2009	21	8 years	100%

* Rates of infection eradication

Table 2. Results of two-stage knee revision arthroplasty

In our series of 43 patients with infected TKA, with characteristic 50% rate of infection with Staphylococcal strains [7], twenty patients underwent a one-stage procedure and 21 patients underwent a two-stage procedure. Our overall data indicate 83% postoperative satisfaction with 87% good and excellent results after revision [41,42]. After an average follow-up of 8 years, subjective satisfaction was reported by 80% of patients without any evidence of re-infection in the whole group of these patients. However in one-stage group a recurrent in-fection was noted in 20% of cases. We use a constrained design of revision prosthesis in order to overcome the expected soft tissue insufficiency in the revised knee (Figure 5).

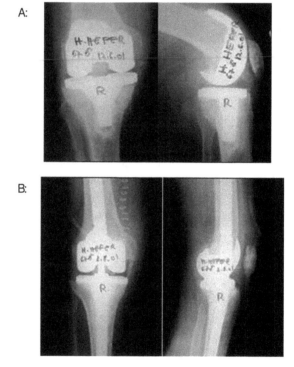

Figure 5. A : Knee radiographs (Anterior-Posterior and Lateral views). Radiolucency is evident around the tibial com-ponent indicating septic loosening. B: Knee radiographs (Anterior-Posterior and Lateral views) following revision with a constrained type prosthesis (CCK).

7. Salvage surgical procedures

In failed treatment of revision TKA or in case of a multioperated knee and a debilitated pa-tient another surgical procedure might be required for limb salvage.

7.1. Knee arthrodesis

Knee arthrodesis should be considered as a therapeutic option when other described above techniques have failed, especially in young patients with high functional demands or in patients with extensive deformities, advanced alterations of the extensor mechanism, deficient soft tissues, immunosuppression or infections by highly virulent bacteria. Arthrodesis provides a stable and pain-free limb. However, there is no flexion and the function of the knee is sacrificed, causing an advanced functional impairment. This is generally an irreversible situation. The procedure can be performed with intramedullary nail, metallic plate or external fixation [43, 44] (Figure 6). We have a good clinical experience using the Ilizarov external fixator for this purpose. We used this method in twelve consecutive patients following failed revision TKA surgery performed as treatment for infected initial knee prosthesis. Solid fusion was achieved in all patients within an average healing time of 27.6 weeks. Average shortening of the affected lib was 3.7 cm. We concluded that the Ilizarov fixator for knee arthrodesis after failed TKR produced favorable results and should be considered for the use by surgeons who are familiar with this technique [44]. The success is dependent on the proficiency of the surgeons in Ilizarov method and patient cooperation.

A: B: C: D:

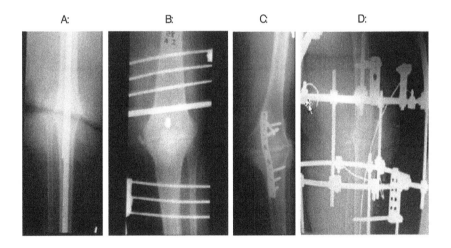

Figure 6. Radiographs of fused knees, following failed revision of TKA, by: A: Intramedullary nail, B: Tubular external fixator. C: Internal fixation by plate and screws, D: Ilizarov external fixator.

7.2. Resection arthroplasty

By this salvage method a permanent removal of the implant and cement with local debridement, without re-implantation, are performed. The purpose of this technique is to create a false joint that may allow a certain range of motion. The leg is immobilized for a period between 3 and 6 months in order to allow the soft tissues retraction with creation of free area for movement with a certain degree of stability. Candidates for this type of treatment are patients with low functional demands [45].

7.3. Limb amputation

This technique should be considered the last resort when dealing with salvage of a prosthetic infection. Its indications are as follows: an uncontrolled infection that threatens the patient's life, large bone loss and severe soft tissue defects [46]. Functional results tend to be extremely poor and patients often end up in a wheelchair. However a successful above knee amputation may provide the best function for patients who otherwise would have a functionless knee joint. In the past limb amputation was required most frequently in infected TKA with cemented stem hinges.

8. Future: Prosthetic design "tuned" to prevention of periprosthetic infection

The best solution is to prevent infection rather than treat it. Nowadays the trend is to design an implant that is less susceptible to infection by using surfaces that will be resistant to bacterial adhesion and generation of biofilm. These designs will be appropriate to prevent infection originating via hematogeous spread. Another approach is to use local slowly released antibacterial agents, such as antibiotics or chemical free radicals, that will keep an efficient periprosthetic high concentration antimicrobial milieu in order to prevent biofilm bacterial masking [47]. This is a very important factor since the effective concentration of antibiotics for penetration of biofilm masking should be 1000 times higher than can be achieved following they usual oral or parenteral administration.

Most of the efforts for generation of anti-biofilm surfaces of the prostheses are still in development stage and still have not gain wide clinical use. Currently three main directions are utilized for this purpose. The most common method is to use titanium surfaces that release bactericidal superoxide radicals [48]. This method is especially appealing since TiO_2 is has no significant cytotoxic effect on mammalian cells. We observed that human osteoblast-like cells in culture remain viable after exposure to high concentration of TiO_2 0.1 mm granules in culture media (10% v:v). Another metal that has bactericidal properties is silver. There are a lot of efforts in designing prosthetic surfaces containing silver [48]. We found that it has a bactericidal effect on different *Staphylococci* strains, but *Pseudomonas aeruginosa* remained resistant to its high concentration (10% v:v). The main problem with the use of silver for prosthetic coating is its toxicity to the host cells. We observed a profound cytotoxic effect in cultures of human osteoblast-like cells exposed to 0.1 mm granules of silver in culture media in bactericidal concentration. For this reason the surfaces coated by TiO_2 have a better bactericidal potential for clinical use.

There is also a possibility to use immobilized antibiotic coverage for prosthetic surfaces. This method is still has not reached a proved clinical use [48].

Currently the widespread method of prosthetic fixation with methyl methacrylate bone cement, containing broad spectrum antibiotics, is the only proven way to create an antimicrobial periprosthetic surrounding. The uncontrolled release of the antibiotics and potential reduced fixation characteristics of the cement containing antibiotics are the main disadvantage of this method, but it is no clinical evidence that might support these concerns.

9. Conclusion

Despite considerable advances in surgical techniques and preoperative care, a 0.5-2% prevalence of infection in total knee arthroplasty (TKA) still poses a great challenge in the treatment of this devastating and costly complication. Current solutions to treat periprosthetic infection remain imperfect. Treatment strategy varies from conservative life-long antibiotic suppression therapy in the very high risk patient, arthroscopic or surgical debridement, revision in one or two-stage, arthrodesis or resection arthroplasty as a salvage procedure, and amputation in life-threatening conditions. The decision on the best method of treatment should be personalized to the patient's general health, the severity of the infection and the complexity of the surgery. Currently most of the surgeons have adopted the two-stage protocol, where prosthetic removal, debridement and culture-specific I.V. therapy prior to re-implantation are regarded as standards of care. Although one-stage revision procedure is practiced by some, there is no clear evidence to define when this procedure can be safely applied, because there is no sufficient reliable data on a clinical reliability of this approach. The quest to perform one-stage revision should be continued, as two-stage operations classify the patient in a multiple operations category, with all the resulting potential complications, such as arthrodesis and amputation. Nevertheless, the threat of re-infection after the one-stage procedure surpasses the potential benefits. Judicious selection of patients is the key for successful mode of treatment. Currently the two-stage exchange arthroplasty, with all its inherent problems and drawbacks, allows only a partial success in treatment of TKA infection. New modalities or avenues for treatment of prosthetic infection are desirable.

Author details

Michael Soudry[1*], Arnan Greental[2], Gabriel Nierenberg[2], Mazen Falah[2] and Nahum Rosenberg[2]

*Address all correspondence to: michael.soudry@gmail.com

1 Department of Orthopaedic Surgery, Hillel Yaffe Medical Center, Hadera, Israel

2 Rambam Health Care Campus, Dept of Orthopaedic Surgery. Haifa, Israel

References

[1] Zimmerli W., Trampuz A., Ochsner PE. Prosthetic-joint infections. N Engl J Med 2004;351(16):1645-54.

[2] Kurtz SM., Ong KL., Lau E., Bozic KJ., Berry D., Parvizi J. Prosthetic joint infection risk after TKA in the Medicare population. Clin Orthop Relate Res 2010: 468(1):52-56.

[3] Bengtson S., Knutson K. The infected knee arthroplasty. A 6-year follow-up of 357 cases. Acta Orthop Scand 1991; 62(4): 301-11.

[4] Hansen AD., Rand JA. Evaluation and treatment of the infection at the site of a total hip and knee arthroplasry. Instr Course Lect 1999;48:111-122.

[5] Ellenrieder et al. Two-stage revision of implant-associated infections after total hip and knee arthroplasty. GMS Krankenhaushygiene Interdisziplinar 2011;6(1):1-8.

[6] Chiang ER et al. Comparison of articulating and static spacers regarding infection with resistant organisms in total knee arthroplasty .Acta Orthopaedica 2011; 82(4): 460-64.

[7] Peel TN., Buising KL., Choong PFM. Prosthetic joint infection: challenges of diagnosis and treatment. ANZ J Surg ;81: 32-39.

[8] Fey PD., Olson ME. Current concepts in biofilm formation of Staphylococcus epidermidis. Future Microbiol 2010 5(6): 917-933.

[9] Sendi P., Zimmerli W. Challenges in periprosthetic knee-joint infection. Int J Artif Organs 2011; 34(9):947-956.

[10] Schafroth M., Zimmerli W., Brunazzi M., Ochsner PE. Infections. In: Ochsner PE ed. Total hip replacement . Berlin: Springer Verlag; 2003. p65-90.

[11] Zimmerli W., Trampuz A., Ochsner PE. Prosthetic-joint infections. N Engl J Med 2004;351(16):1645-54.

[12] Giuleri SG., Graber P., Ochsner PE., Zimmerli W. Management of infection associated with THA according to a treatment algorithm. Infection; 2004; 32(4):222-8.

[13] Smith SL., Wastle ML., Forster I. Radiolonuclide bone scintigraphy in the detection of significant complications after total knee joint replacement. Clin Radiol; 2001: 56: 221-4.

[14] Hain SF., O'Doherty MJ., Smith MA. Functional imaging and the orthopedic surgeon. J. Bone Joint Surg Br. 2002; 84:315-21.

[15] Shih LY., Wu JJ., Yang DJ. Erythrocyte sedimentation rate and CRP values with THA. Clinic Orthop 1987:225:238-46.

[16] Di Cesare PE., Chang E., Preston CF., Liu CJ. Serum Interleukin-6 as a Marker of Periprosthetic Infection Following Total Hip and Knee Arthroplasty. J Bone Joint Surg Am 2005; 87(9):1921-1927.

[17] Marian BD., Martin DS., Levine MJ., Booth RE., Tuan RS. Polymerase Chain. Reaction Detection of Bacterial Infection in Total Knee Arthroplasty. Clinical Orthop 1996; 331: 11-22.

[18] Trampuz A., Piper K., Jacobson M. et al. Sonication of removed hip and knee prostheses for diagnosis of infection. N Engl J Med 2007;357:654-63.

[19] Tampuz A., Hansen AD., Osmon DR., Mandrekar J., Steckekberg JM., Patel R. Advances in the laboratory diagnosis of prosthetic joint infection. Rev Med Microbiol 2003; 14:1-14.

[20] Parvizi J., Della Valle CJ. In: AAOS Clinical Practice Guideline. Diagnosis and Treatment of periprosthetic joint infections of the hip and knee. J. Am Acad Orthop Surg 2010;18:771-772.

[21] Grogan TJ., Dorey F., Rollins J. et al. Deep sepsis following TKA. JBJS A, 1986: 68:226-234.

[22] Johnson DP., Bannister GC. The outcome of infected arthoplasty of the knee. JBJS B 1986:68;289-291.

[23] Do CSO., Beauchamp CP., Clarke HD., Spangehl MJ. A Two-stage Retention Debridement Protocol for Acute Periprosthetic joint infection. Clin Orthop Relat Res. 2010: Aug;468(8):2029-38.

[24] Parvizi J., Ghanem E., Sharkey P. Prosthetic Joint Infections. Clin Orthop Relat Res 2007; 461:44-47.

[25] Coventry MB., Beckenbaugh RD., Nolan DR., Ilstrup DM. 2,012 total hip arthroplasties. A study of postoperative course and early complications. J Bone Joint Surg Am. 1974;56(2):273-84.

[26] Parkinson RW., Kay PR., Rawal A. A case for one-stage revision in infected totalknee arthroplasty. Knee 2011; 18:1–4.

[27] Buechel FF. The Infected Total Knee Arthroplasty. Just When You Thought It Was Over. The Journal of Arthroplasty 2004; Suppl 4: 19.

[28] Fink B., Gebhard A., Fuerst M., Berger I., Schafer P. High Diagnostic Value of Synovial Biopsy in Periprosthetic Joint Infection of the Hip. Clin Orthop Relat Res. in press.

[29] Nickinson RS.J, Board TN., Gambhir AK., Porter ML., Kay PR. Two stage revision knee arthroplasty for infection with massive bone loss. A technique to achieve spacer stability. Knee 2012;19: 24–27.

[30] Kohl S., Evangelopoulos DS., Kohlhof H., Krueger A., Hartel M., Roeder C., Eggli S. An intraoperatively moulded PMMA prostheses-like spacer for two-stage revision of infected total knee arthroplasty. Knee 2011;18: 464–469.

[31] Choi HR., Malchau H., Bedair H. Are Prosthetic Spacers Safe to Use in 2-Stage Treatment for Infected Total Knee Arthroplasty? J of Arthroplasty 2012; in press.

[32] Macmull S., Bartlett W., Miles GW., Blunn J., Pollock RC., Carrington RWJ., Skinner JA., Cannon SR., Briggs TWR. Custom-made hinged spacers in revision knee surgery for patients with infection, bone loss and instability. Knee 2010;17: 403–406.

[33] Joseph TN., Chen AL., Di Cesare PE. Use of antibiotic-impregnated cement in total joint arthroplasty. J Am Acad Orthop Surg 2003;11:38-47.

[34] Hanssen AD., Rand JA. Evaluation and treatment of infection at the site of a total hip or knee arthroplasty. J Bone Joint Surg 1998; 80:910-922.

[35] Hoad-Reddick DA., Evans CR., Norman .P, Stockly I. Is there a role for extended antibiotic therapy in a two-stage revision of the infected knee arthroplasty?. J Bone Joint Surg Br 2005; 87-B:171-174.

[36] Freeman MA., Sudlow RA., Casewell MW., Radcliff SS. The management of infected total knee replacements. J Bone Joint Surg Br 1985; 67:764-768.

[37] Haleem AA., Berry DJ., Hanssen AD. Mid-term to long-term follow-up of two-stage reimplantation for infected total knee arthroplasty. Clin Orthop. 2004: 428:35-39.

[38] Wilde AH., Ruth JT. Two-stage reimplantation in infected total knee arhroplasty. Clin Orthop 1988; 236:23-35.

[39] Von Foerster G., Klüber D., Kähler U. Mid- to long-term results after treatment of 118 cases of periprosthetic infections after knee joint replacement using one-stage exchange surgery]. Orthopade. 1991 Jun;20(3):244-52.

[40] Windsor R., Insall J. Management of the infected total knee arthroplasty. In: Insall-Scott, eds. Surgery of the Knee. 1st ed. Churchill Livingstone, New York, 1983. 959-974.

[41] Soudry M., Greental A., Niereberg G., Falah M. One and two-stage revision in infected TKA. JBJS B. 2005: Vol 87-B. Supp III: 389.

[42] Soudry M., Nierenberg G., Msika C., Jontschew DA., Falah M. One vs two-stage revision of infected knee arthroplasty. Portugese Journal of Orthopaedics. 2009: Vol 17 (4): 1-11.

[43] Klinger HM., Spahn G., Schultz W., Baums MH. Arthrodesis of the knee after failed infected total knee arthroplasty. Knee Surg Sports Traumatol Arthrosc.2006; 14(5): 447-53.

[44] David R., Shtarker H., Horesh Z., Tsur A., Soudry M. Knee Arthrodesis with the Ilizarov after failed knee arthroplasty. Orthopedics, 2001 Jan: 24(1):33-6.

[45] Falahee MH., Matthews LS., Kaufer H. Resection Arthroplasty as a salvage procedure for a knee with infection after TKA. JBJS A 1987: 69: 1013-1021.

[46] Pring DJ., Marks, Angel JC. Mobility after amputation for failed knee replacement. JBJS B 1988: 70: 770-771).

[47] Vasilev K., Cook .J, Griesser HJ. Antibacterial surfaces for biomedical devices. Expert Rev Med Devices 2009; 6(5): 553-567.

[48] Visai L., De Nardo L., Punta C., Melone L., Cigada A., Imbriani M., Arciala CR. Titanium oxide antibacterial surfaces in biomedical devices. Int J Artif Organs 2011; 34(9):929-946.

[49] Lu H., Kou B., Lin J. One-stage reimplantation for the salvage of total knee arthroplasty complicated by infection. Zhonghua Wai Ke Za Zhi. 1997 Aug;35(8):456-8.

[50] Siegel A., Frommelt L., Runde W. Therapy of bacterial knee joint infection by radical synovectomy and implantation of a cemented stabilized knee joint endoprosthesis. Chirurg. 2000 Nov;71(11):1385-91.

[51] Hanssen AD., Rand JA., Osmon DR. Treatment of the infected total knee arthroplasty with insertion of another prosthesis. The effect of antibiotic-impregnated bone cement. Clin Orthop Relat Res. 1994 Dec;(309):44-55.

[52] Goldman RT., Scuderi GR., Insall JN. 2-stage reimplantation for infected total knee replacement. Clin Orthop Relat Res. 1996 Oct;(331):118-24.

[53] Gacon G., Laurencon M., Van de Velde D., Giudicelli DP. Two stages reimplantation for infection after knee arthroplasty. Apropos of a series of 29 cases. Rev Chir Orthop Reparatrice Appar Mot. 1997;83(4):313-23.

[54] Hirakawa K., Stulberg BN., Wilde AH., Bauer TW., Secic M. Results of two-stage reimplantation for infected total knee arthroplasty. J Arthroplasty. 1998 Jan;13(1):22-8.

[55] Siebel T., Kelm J., Porsch M., Regitz T., Neumann WH. Two-stage exchange of infected knee arthroplasty with a prosthesis-like interim cement spacer. Acta Orthop Belg. 2002 Apr;68(2):150-6.

[56] Pietsch M., Wenisch C., Traussnig S., Trnoska R., Hofmann S. Temporary articulating spacer with antibiotic-impregnated cement for an infected knee endoprosthesis. Orthopade. 2003 Jun;32(6):490-7.

Chapter 8

Management of Prosthetic Infection According to Organism

Trisha Peel, Kirsty Buising, Michelle Dowsey and
Peter Choong

Additional information is available at the end of the chapter

1. Introduction

Since the advent of prosthetic joint replacement surgery, patients with arthritis have had significant improvement in pain-relief, mobility and quality of life. Approximately 90,000 Australians undergo joint replacement surgery each year [1]. With an ageing population, this number will increase (figure 1). Similar data from USA predicts that by 2030 the number of procedures per year will increase to 4.05 million [2]. Despite the overall success of this surgery, infection of the prosthesis remains a devastating complication [3]. Of concern, the incidence of prosthetic joint infection is increasing, in proportion to the number of procedures being performed [4]. Significant patient morbidity is associated with prosthetic joint infections, including the need for further operative procedures, long-term antibiotic therapy with associated toxicity, and prolonged hospitalisation [3]. In addition, the cost to the health system is substantial. The cost of treating infection is 3-5 times the cost of primary arthroplasty [5, 6]. In Australia, the annual additional expenditure incurred as a result of this devastating complication is estimated at AUD $90 million per year [6]. In the United States, the annual cost of treatment of prosthetic joint infection is projected to exceed US$1.6 billion dollars by 2020[7].

The incidence of prosthetic joint infection is estimated at 1-3% of all prosthetic joint replacements [3]. In prosthetic hip replacement, the rate of infection is estimated at 0.88% and in knee replacement at 0.92%[4]. The incidence of prosthetic joint infections is higher for upper limb arthroplasty; in shoulders the incidence of infection is 1.8-4% and in elbow replacements the incidence of infection is 3-7.5% of patients [8-10].

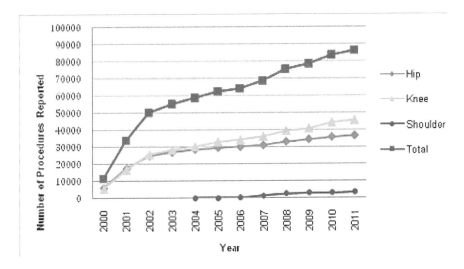

Figure 1. Prosthetic Joint Replacement Surgery in Australia *(adapted from AOA National Joint Replacement Registry[1])*

A number of pre-operative factors have been implicated in the development of prosthetic joint infection, including revision arthroplasty, diabetes mellitus and rheumatoid arthritis [11-16]. The risk factors for prosthetic joint infection differ according to the joint replaced. Obesity plays a greater role in the evolution of prosthetic joint infection in lower limb arthroplasty [17-19]. The presence of post-operative wound complications, including high drain tube losses, wound discharge and superficial surgical site infection have been implicated as risk factors for development of prosthetic joint infection in hip and knee arthroplasty[11, 20]. In addition the presence of a drain tube appears to be protective for prosthetic knee infections [17, 18]. Underlying inflammatory arthritis and concomitant steroid use increases the risk of infections in all arthroplasty surgery but the association is particularly marked in the upper limb [16, 17]. In addition male gender has been identified as a risk factor in shoulder arthroplasty infection, potentially through the interaction with *Propionibacterium acnes* (see below)[12].

2. Pathogenesis

There are two main mechanisms of acquisition of prosthetic joint infection; (i) direct inoculation of the prosthesis at the time of surgery or with manipulation of the joint and (ii) seeding from the blood stream at a later time[3]. The pathogenesis of prosthetic joint infections differs to that of many other bacterial infections through the property of microorganisms to form biofilms[3]. Microorganisms can exist in two phenotypic forms: the planktonic form which is encountered in the majority of acute bacterial infections such as bacterial septicaemia or pneumonia, and the sessile form associated with medical device infections such as prosthetic joint infections[21]. In medical device associated infections, the planktonic bacteria seed the device and undergo a phenotypic change transforming into the sessile bacteria. The biofilm is comprised of the sessile bacteria and the extracellular matrix they secrete[21]. This matrix protects the microorganisms from antibiotics and the host immune response and is thought to be the underlying reason for persistence of infections[21].

3. Microbiology

Staphylococcus aureus and coagulase negative Staphylococcus species are the most common aetiological agents of prosthetic joint infections. The incidence of methicillin resistant strains such as methicillin resistant *Staphylococcus aureus* (MRSA) differ globally; the rate of MRSA prosthetic joint infections across Europe and the Americans MRSA ranges from 8% to 30%[22-24]. In Australia, 26% of prosthetic joint infections are due to MRSA. In addition, methicillin resistant coagulase negative Staphylococci account for a further 22% of isolates [25, 26].

Gram negative bacilli such as *Escherichia coli* and *Pseudomonas aeruginosa* are the next most common isolates[3, 26]. Other microorganisms such as enterococci, streptococci, corynebacterium, fungal species and mycobacterial species are reported less commonly [3, 27]. Of note, the microbiology of prosthetic joint infection differs between upper limb and lower limb arthroplasty: *Propionibacterium acnes* is one of the most common microorganisms encountered in shoulder prosthetic joint infection, occurring in up to 40% of shoulder arthroplasty infections [16, 28, 29]. This association may be due to the increased occurrence of *Propionibacterium acnes* around the head and neck, in particular in the sebaceous glands and hair bulbs [12].

From a review of 6,282 prosthetic hip and knee replacements performed at St Vincent's Hospital Melbourne (SVHM) between 2000 and 2012, there were 138 definite infections (table 1). Prosthetic joint infection was defined by the typical diagnostic criteria which include those discussed further in table 2. Microorganisms were defined as the causative pathogen/s if isolated on two or more intra-operative specimens.

The microbiology of hip and knee prosthetic joint infection was similar, except for an increased number of culture negative infections in prosthetic knee joints and increased isolation of *Enterococcus faecalis* from prosthetic hip infections. From SVHM data there was an increased rate of incisional surgical site infections in knee arthroplasties that later developed prosthetic joint infections compared to hip arthroplasty (28% versus 12%)[17, 30]. Therefore it is postulated that the increased number of culture negative infections in the knee replacement patients may reflect increased antibiotic exposure for superficial wound complications or for unrecognised prosthetic joint infection.

	Number (%) of Prosthetic Knee Infections (n=66)	Number (%) of Prosthetic Hip Infections (n=72)	Number (%) of All Prosthetic Joint Infections (n=138)
Gram positive organisms	48 (73%)	60 (83%)	108 (78%)
Staphylococcus aureus	25 (38%)	35 (49%)	60 (43%)
Methicillin sensitive	16 (24%)	17 (24%)	33 (24%)
Methicillin resistant	9 (14%)	18 (25%)	27 (20%)
CNS	14 (21%)	13 (18%)	26 (19%)
Methicillin sensitive	1 (2%)	0	1 (1%)
Methicillin resistant	13 (20%)	13 (18%)	26 (19%)
Streptococcus species	4 (6%)	2 (3%)	6 (4%)
Enterococcus faecalis	4 (6%)	10 (14%)	14 (10%)
Other gram positive organisms*	3 (5%)	1 (1%)	4 (3%)
Gram negative organisms	9 (14%)	14 (19%)	23 (17%)
Escherichia coli	1 (2%)	3 (4%)	4 (3%)
Morganella morganii	4 (6%)	0	4 (3%)
Klebsiella pneumoniae	0	1 (1%)	1 (1%)
Serratia marcescens	2 (3%)	0	2 (1%)
Pseudomonas aeruginosa	0	1 (1%)	1 (1%)
Citrobacter koseri	0	1 (1%)	1 (1%)
Enterobacter cloacae	0	3 (4%)	3 (2%)
Proteus mirabilis	2 (3%)	4 (6%)	6 (4%)
Bacteroides fragilis	0	1 (1%)	1 (1%)
Culture negative	17 (26%)	11 (15%)	28 (20%)

CNS = Coagulase negative Staphylococcus species

* Other gram positive isolates included 1 Peptostreptococcus species, 1 Bacillus cereus and 2 Corynebacterium species

Table 1. Microbiology of 138 prosthetic hip and knee joint infections seen at SVHM between 2000 and 2012

4. Clinical classification and presentation

Prosthetic joint infections are classified as (i) early (developing in the first three months after implantation), (ii) delayed (occurring 3 to 24 months after surgery) and (iii) late (greater than 24 months) or (iv) haematagenous [3]. Haematogenous seeding of the prosthesis typically occur late (after 24 months) but can occur at any time point following implantation [3, 31].

The clinical manifestation differs according to time of presentation. In early prosthetic joint infection, patients typically present with surgical wound complications such as purulent discharge, erythema and swelling of the affected joint (Figure 2) [3, 32]. In delayed and late infections, pain is the predominant feature with patients reporting a history of slowly increasing pain involving the prosthetic joint [32]. Haematogenous infections in contrast, typically are associated with a history of a joint that was free of any problems for several months to years before an acute onset of fever, erythema around the surgical wound and pain in the affected joint[33].

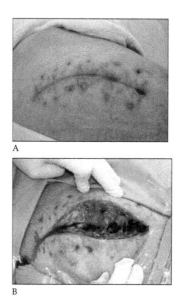

Figure 2. Early Prosthetic Hip Joint Infection (A) at presentation with infection showing wound erythema, swelling and purulent discharge and (B) intra-operative appearance showing purulence surrounding the prosthetic joint.

The presentation of shoulder arthroplasty infection due to *Propionibacterium* acnes is generally delayed or late[12]. The classic features of infection are frequently absent with pain and stiffness of the joint the predominant symptoms [12, 34]. Bruising along the surgical wound has been described as a pathognomonic sign of *Propionibacterium acnes* shoulder arthroplasty infection [34].

5. Diagnosis of prosthetic joint infections

The diagnosis of infections is challenging due to the absence of an internationally accepted gold standard for defining arthroplasty infection. Current definitions rely on a number of parameters including clinical, microbiological and histopathological features (Table 2) [3, 35-39].

Prompt recognition and diagnosis of prosthetic joint infection is imperative to minimize patient suffering and to improve patient outcomes [40]. Isolation of the causative microorganism is the most important diagnostic test as it allows confirmation of diagnosis and assessment of antimicrobial susceptibilities. Infection of the prosthesis is suggested by the isolation of the same microorganism from 2 or more intra-operative specimens [3, 35, 36] To increase the likelihood of diagnosis, ≥5 peri-prosthetic tissue specimens should be obtained intra-operatively with each specimen placed in separate sterile containers [35, 36]. This is of particular importance for skin commensals such as *Propionibacterium acnes* and coagulase negative Staphylococcus species to aid in distinguishing true infection from specimen contamination.

The diagnosis of prosthetic joint infection should be considered in patients with any of the following [3, 36-39]:

Presence of peri-prosthetic purulence observed intra-operatively; OR

Isolation of indistinguishable micro-organism/s on ≥2 intra-operative specimens (tissue or joint aspirate cultures); OR

Presence of a sinus tract in communication with the prosthetic joint; OR

Histopathological features of acute infections with ≥5 neutrophils per-high power field (x 500 magnifications) in 5 different microscopic fields.

Table 2. Diagnosis of Prosthetic Joint Infection

Prior exposure to antibiotic therapy increases the risk of culture negative prosthetic joint infection [30, 37, 41]. Therefore antibiotic therapy should not be commenced until after obtaining multiple intra-operative specimens, except in the case of the septic patient in whom commencement of antibiotic therapy should not be delayed. In patients with delayed and late infections, who have received antibiotic therapy prior to obtainment of intra-operative cultures, definitive surgery may be delayed for 2-4 weeks after cessation of antibiotics to increase the intra-operative yield[30, 37, 41].

Sonication of the explanted prosthesis disrupts the biofilm and may increase the diagnostic yield of microbiological culture. Sonication is particularly useful in patients who have received antibiotics in 14 days preceding surgery [37]. Prolongation of microbiological cultures from 3 to 14 days also increases the diagnostic yield, particularly of more fastidious organisms such as *Propionibacterium acnes* [42].

6. Management of prosthetic joint infection

The goal of treatment of prosthetic joint infection is to eradicate the biofilm dwelling microorganisms, whilst maintaining function of the joint and patient quality of life[3].

The surgical strategies to manage prosthetic joint infection include: (i) one-stage or two-stage exchange procedures, (ii) debridement and retention of the prosthesis in conjunction with biofilm active antibiotics, (iii) removal of the prosthesis +/- arthrodesis, (iv) amputation of the affected limb and (v) chronic suppression without surgical debridement of the infected joint. Removal of the prosthesis and amputation are associated with significant impairment of mobility. Chronic suppression is association with a high rate of recurrence of infection. Therefore these strategies are reserved for patients with significant co-morbidities or in patients with recalcitrant infection [3, 33]. Exchange procedures and debridement and retention are the two strategies that best meet the goals of treatment [3, 33].

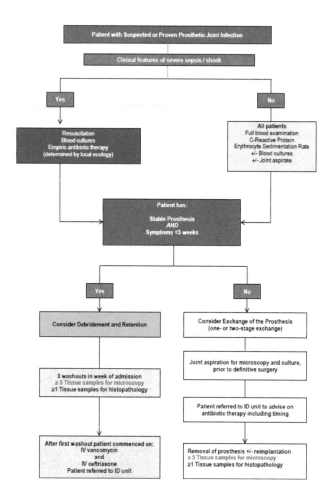

Figure 3. SVHM Protocol Algorithm for Management of Prosthetic Joint Infection

Given the heterogeneous nature of prosthetic joint infections there are no large randomized control trials to guide recommendations. Surgical strategies differ significantly worldwide; exchange procedures are the favoured treatment modality in Northern America, whereas debridement and retention is more commonly performed in Australia and parts of Europe [3, 26, 33]. A number of treatment algorithms exist to guide management decisions and these are based on factors such as duration of symptoms, the stability of implant, patient co-morbidities and the type of infecting microorganism[3, 33]. Compared to the exchange procedures, patients managed with debridement and retention of the implant undergo fewer and less extensive surgical procedures and have shorter duration of hospitalisation and immobilisation [3, 33, 43]. Therefore early and haematogenous infections can be managed by debridement and retention. However, if the implant is loose, if the duration of symptoms prior to presentation exceed 21 days or if the isolated pathogen is resistant to biofilm-active antibiotics, the likelihood of treatment success for debridement and retention is markedly reduced[3, 33]. Therefore if the patient has any of the above features, expert opinion recommends patients undergo prosthesis exchange (either as a one-stage or two-stage procedure). Delayed or late prosthetic joint infections should be managed by one- or two-stage exchange; debridement and retention of the prosthesis in this setting is associated with a high failure rate[3, 33].

At SVHM, a management protocol was established through collaboration between the Orthopaedic and Infectious Diseases Departments. The abbreviated algorithm is shown in Figure 3. The antibiotic regimens for different pathogens are detailed in Table 3. At SVHM patients managed by debridement and retention of the prosthesis undergo 3 debridements of the infected joint. The liner is changed, where feasible, but other mobile parts are not routinely changed. This differs from other protocols for debridement and retention, in which patients undergo a single debridement with exchange of all mobile parts and liners [33]. Regardless of technique, the aim of the debridement/s is to reduce the microbial burden prior to instigation of antibiotic therapy with activity against the biofilm-dwelling microorganisms.

7. Staphylococcus aureus and coagulase negative Staphylococcus species

Rifampicin has excellent activity against Staphylococcal biofilms and is the mainstay of treatment in these infections, particularly with debridement and retention [3, 33, 44-46]. Older treatment algorithms recommended against debridement and retention for MRSA however, emerging evidence suggests that this is a suitable strategy in carefully selected patients [33, 46, 47].

Staphylococcus becomes rapidly resistant to rifampicin if this antibiotic is used alone, therefore rifampicin must always be administered with a second agent (companion drug) [48]. Fluoroquinolones, such as ciprofloxacin, are frequently used as companion drugs however fluoroquinolone resistance is increasing thus limiting the utility of this combination[25]. Alternate companion drugs for rifampicin include fusidic acid, trimethoprim-sulfamethoxazole, minocycline, daptomycin and linezolid [33, 47-52]. There are no clinical studies comparing the efficacy of different drugs used in combination with rifampicin. In Australia including SVHM, fusidic acid is commonly prescribed as a companion drug for rifampicin [47] [26].

Rifampicin based regimens are recommended even for methicillin sensitive isolates. Given the high oral bioavailability of rifampicin, a move to oral therapy is suggested as soon as the patient can reliably take oral diet after completion of surgical debridements. For those few patients who are bacteraemic, however, more prolonged intravenous therapy may be required along with appropriate investigation to exclude other foci of infection, such as endocarditis.

In patients with MRSA infections managed with two-stage exchange; the insertion of a spacer should be avoided as there is an increased rate of treatment failure [3, 33, 53]. In addition, an association between the presence of a spacer and the development of rifampicin resistance in MRSA strains has been reported [53].

8. Streptococcus

Streptococcus are the causative agent in 8% of prosthetic joint infections[26]. In general the treatment outcomes are excellent for all surgical strategies for Streptococcal arthroplasty infection [54-58]. However, the outcomes with group B streptococcal infections are mixed with some studies reporting poorer outcomes with these isolates [58-60]. In general intravenous benzylpenicillin or ceftriaxone can be used (often for 2 weeks) before a shift to high dose oral amoxicillin. In some circumstances, with typable streptococci where susceptibility to rifampicin is expected, rifampicin can be added to the amoxicillin as part of the oral regimen although the evidence for this practice is still not clear.

9. Enterococcus

Enterococcus is an uncommon cause of prosthetic joint infection however, the incidence of these infections is increasing[61]. At our institution, *Enterococcus faecalis* was isolated in 10% of all infections. It is a common isolate in polymicrobial infections of the prosthetic hip joint. There are little published data to guide treatment of enterococcal prosthetic joint infection. Some experts recommend treatment strategies extrapolated from other enterococcal infections, in particular enterococcal endocarditis [61]. Beta-lactam antibiotics, such as penicillin are bacteriostatic against enterococci, therefore combination therapy with aminoglycosides such as gentamicin, is recommended for management of enterococcal endocarditis[62]. However data from retrospective studies suggest there is no additional benefit with combination therapy with aminoglycosides in enterococcal prosthetic joint infections and, of great concern, there was significant nephrotoxicity and ototoxicity associated with aminoglycoside therapy[61]. Euba et al examined the role of ampicillin-ceftriaxone combination therapy, however, only 3 patients with enterococcal prosthetic joint infection were included in this study and 2 of those patients had late infections[63]. Therefore the role of this combination therapy remains unclear and further studies are required. Recent in-vitro models have suggested rifampicin in combination either with ciprofloxacin or linezolid are the most efficacious antibiotic combinations against biofilm dwelling Enterococcus faecalis, although there are no reports at present of the use of these combinations in patients[64].

Enterococcus faecium is infrequently involved in prosthetic joint infections; however, it presents significant treatment challenges, owing to increased resistance when compared to *Enterococcus* faecalis. In particular, *Enterococcus faecium* is increasingly resistant to benzylpenicillin and amoxicillin[62]. There is little clinical data outlining management approaches for *Enterococcus faecium*, however, exchange procedures are likely to be the optimal strategy in these infections. Other resistant enterococcal prosthetic joint infection including vancomycin resistant enterococcus (VRE), also are very uncommon. In a statewide review of 163 prosthetic joint infections, VRE was isolated once (0.6%). Two-stage exchange of the prosthesis is recommended for VRE arthroplasty infections in conjunction with agents such as daptomycin, linezolid or pristinamycin. In all enterococcal infections, including VRE, the use of spacers in two-stage exchange procedures is not recommended due to the increased risk of treatment failure [3, 33].

10. Gram negative bacilli

For gram-negative bacilli infections, ciprofloxacin has been shown to be effective in guinea pig tissue cage models[65]. There is conflicting data on the clinical outcomes of gram-negative bacilli infections, particularly with debridement and retention. The reported success rate for debridement and retention ranges from 27%-94% with a similar range reported for exchange procedures [66-70]. The likelihood of success may relate to the quality of the debridement and meticulous care should be taken to ensure removal of all dead and devitalised tissue and removal of all cement in the exchange procedures [69]. In addition, gram-negative bacteria, particularly *Pseudomonas aeruginosa*, have a propensity to develop resistance to fluoroquinolones in-vivo[62]. In light of this, many experts recommend a 2-4 week course of beta-lactam antibiotic prior to commencement of ciprofloxacin to reduce the bacterial load and thus reduce the likelihood of generation of in-vivo resistance [33].

11. Propionibacterium

As with all other infections, the duration of symptoms dictates the most appropriate surgical strategy for *Propionibacterium acnes* prosthetic joint infection. In *Propionibacterium* arthroplasty infection, the majority of cases are delayed or late presentations, with a long duration of symptoms[12]. Therefore prosthesis exchange is the surgical modality of choice.

Evidence of the ability of *Propionibacterium acnes* to form biofilms is emerging. A number of in-vitro models have been developed to assess the activity of antibiotics against biofilm-associated *Propionibacterium*. As with staphylococcal biofilm models, the activity of rifampicin is preserved with *Propionibacterium* biofilms[71]. The emergence of rifampicin resistance with monotherapy has not been demonstrated[71]. In one study combination therapy with daptomycin and rifampicin was the most effective treatment regimen[71]. Other studies have demonstrated penicillin alone or combination therapy with rifampicin and linezolid are also effective against *Propionibacterium* biofilms[72].

The antibiotic regimens reported to treat patients with *Propionibacterium acnes* prosthetic joint infection are diverse and include: penicillin, amoxicillin, ceftriaxone, clindamycin and rifampicin-fluoroquinolone or rifampicin-clindamycin combination therapy [73, 74]. In general, we recommend IV benzylpenicillin followed by high dose oral amoxicillin combined with rifampicin.

12. Fungi

Fungal prosthetic joint infections are rare. The majority of fungal prosthetic joint infections are due to Candida species however, other fungal species have been reported including Aspergillus species, *Cryptococcus neoformans*, Zygomycetes, *Histoplasma capsulatum, Rhodotorula minuta* [75-78] (figure 4).

The results for debridement and retention and exchange procedures for management of fungal prosthetic joint are poor. In treatment guidelines from the Infectious Diseases Society of America, resection arthroplasty is recommended for prosthetic joint infection due to candidal species[79]. In addition, the use of a spacer following resection of the prosthesis is associated with a high rate of failure and should be avoided [75, 80]. If reimplantation is considered following prosthesis resection, a prolonged period (3-6 months) prior to reinsertion is recommended [81]. Finally, in candidal prosthetic joint infections, there is emerging evidence that the activity of caspofungin is better preserved in the presence of biofilm, compared to fluconazole [80, 82]. For other non candidal fungi, individualized expert advice should be sought to guide antimicrobial choice.

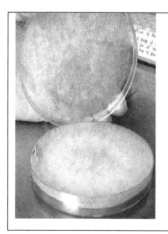

These microbiological cultures were obtained from a patient with disseminated Rhizopus infection including prosthetic hip joint involvement. The patient had significant comorbidities and was managed with debridement and retention of the prosthesis and long-term posaconazole therapy[76].

Figure 4. Rhizopus species cultured from an infected prosthetic hip joint. Photo courtesy of Dr Harsha Sheorey, Microbiology Department, St Vincent's Hospital Melbourne.

13. Culture negative

One of the greatest challenges in management is the 'culture negative' prosthetic joint in-fection. In published case series, the reported rate of culture-negative prosthetic joint in-fection ranges from 5-41% [3, 27, 83]. A number of factors contribute to the failure of microbiological cultures to isolate a pathogen including poor culture technique (including obtaining fewer than 5 intra-operative specimens), fastidious organisms that are difficult to culture and prior antibiotic exposure that impedes bacterial growth. Of these mecha-nisms, prior antibiotic exposure is the most common reason for failing to isolate a causa-tive pathogen. In some studies, 44% of patients with culture negative prosthetic joint infection were receiving antibiotic therapy at the time of obtainment of microbiological specimens[30]. Indeed, the receipt of antibiotics in the 3 months prior to presentation with prosthetic joint infection, lead to a 5-fold increased chance of culture-negative prosthetic joint infection [41].

The choice of antibiotic treatment in culture negative prosthetic joint infection should be guided by local ecology. In addition, if patients had prior exposure to antibiotic therapy, the spectrum of these antibiotics may also influence subsequent antibiotic selection. The results for culture negative prosthetic joint infection are generally similar to culture positive pros-thetic joint infection [41].

14. Conclusion

With an ageing population and the increasing popularity of arthroplasty, prosthetic joint in-fection will continue to present a diagnostic and management challenge to clinicians. Treat-ment approaches for arthroplasty infection are still under debate, in particular, optimal treatment strategy for different microorganisms. Increasing understanding of the role of bio-film in the pathogenesis of prosthetic joint infections and investigation of the activity of dif-ferent antimicrobial agents against biofilm associated microorganisms will provide important information to guide therapy. In addition, multicentre studies and collaborative research groups are key to providing more detailed treatment particularly for less common-ly encountered pathogens.

Author details

Trisha Peel, Kirsty Buising, Michelle Dowsey and Peter Choong

University of Melbourne, St. Vincent's Hospital Melbourne, Australia

References

[1] Australian Orthopaedic Association. National Bone and Joint Registry Annual Report 2011. Adelaide 2011.

[2] Kurtz S, Ong K, Lau E, Mowat F, Halpern M. Projections of primary and revision hip and knee arthroplasty in the United States from 2005 to 2030. Journal of Bone and Joint Surgery 2007;89-A(4):780-5.

[3] Zimmerli W, Trampuz A, Ochsner PE. Prosthetic-joint infections. New England Journal of Medicine. 2004;351(16):1645-54.

[4] Kurtz SM, Lau E, Schmier J, Ong KL, Zhao K, Parvizi J. Infection burden for hip and knee arthroplasty in the United States. Journal of Arthroplasty. 2008;23(7):984-91.

[5] Bozic KJ, Ries MD. The impact of infection after total hip arthroplasty on hospital and surgeon resource utilization. Journal of Bone and Joint Surgery. 2005;87-A(8): 1746-51.

[6] Peel TN, Dowsey MM, Buising KL, Liew D, Choong PF. Cost analysis of debridement and retention for management of prosthetic joint infection. Clinical Microbiology and Infection. 2011;in press.

[7] Kurtz SM, Lau E, Watson H, Schmier JK, Parvizi J. Economic burden of periprosthetic joint infection in the United States. Journal of Arthroplasty. 2012;in press.

[8] Coste JS, Reig S, Trojani C, Berg M, Walch G, Boileau P. The management of infection in arthroplasty of the shoulder. Journal of Bone and Joint Surgery 2004;86-Br(1):65-9.

[9] Vergidis P, Greenwood-Quaintance KE, Sanchez-Sotelo J, Morrey BF, Steinmann SP, Karau MJ, et al. Implant sonication for the diagnosis of prosthetic elbow infection. Journal of Shoulder and Elbow Surgery. 2011;20(8):1275-81.

[10] Achermann Y, Vogt M, Spormann C, Kolling C, Remschmidt C, Wust J, et al. Characteristics and outcome of 27 elbow periprosthetic joint infections: results from a 14-year cohort study of 358 elbow prostheses. Clinical Microbiology and Infection. 2011;17(3):432-8.

[11] Berbari EF, Hanssen AD, Duffy MC, Steckelberg JM, Ilstrup DM, Harmsen WS, et al. Risk factors for prosthetic joint infection: case-control study. Clinical Infectious Diseases. 1998;27(5):1247-54.

[12] Kanafani ZA, Sexton DJ, Pien BC, Varkey J, Basmania C, Kaye KS. Postoperative joint infections due to Propionibacterium species: a case-control study. Clinical Infectious Diseases. 2009;49(7):1083-5.

[13] Poss R, Thornhill TS, Ewald FC, Thomas WH, Batte NJ, Sledge CB. Factors influencing the incidence and outcome of infection following total joint arthroplasty. Clinical Orthopaedics and Related Research. 1984;182:117-.

[14] Bengtson S, Knutson K. The infected knee arthroplasty. Acta Orthopaedica Scandinavica. 1991;62(4):301-11.

[15] Yang K, Yeo SJ, Lee BP, Lo NN. Total knee arthroplasty in diabetic patients: a study of 109 consecutive cases. Journal of Arthroplasty. 2001;16(1):102-6.

[16] Topolski MS, Chin PYK, Sperling JW, Cofield RH. Revision shoulder arthroplasty with positive intraoperative cultures: the value of preoperative studies and intraoperative histology. Journal of Shoulder and Elbow Surgery. 2002;15(4):402-6.

[17] Peel TN, Dowsey MM, Daffy JR, Stanley PA, Choong PF, Buising KL. Risk factors for prosthetic hip and knee infections according to arthroplasty site. Journal of Hospital Infection. 2011;79(2):129-33.

[18] Dowsey MM, Choong PFM. Obese diabetic patients are at substantial risk for deep infection after primary TKA. Clinical Orthopaedics and Related Research. 2009;467(6):1577-81.

[19] Dowsey MM, Choong PF. Obesity is a major risk factor for prosthetic infection after primary hip arthroplasty. Clinical Orthopaedics and Related Research. 2008;466(1): 153-8.

[20] Surin VV, Sundholm K, Backman L. Infection after total hip replacement. With special reference to a discharge from the wound. Journal of Bone and Joint Surgery 1983;65-Br(4):412-8.

[21] Costerton JW. Bacterial biofilms: a common cause of persistent infections. Science. 1999;284(5418):1318-22.

[22] Parvizi J, Ghanem E, Azzam K, Davis E, Jaberi F, Hozack W. Periprosthetic infection: are current treatment strategies adequate? Acta Orthopedica Belgium. 2008;74(6): 793-800.

[23] Pulido L, Ghanem E, Joshi A, Purtill JJ, Parvizi J, Pulido L, et al. Periprosthetic joint infection: the incidence, timing, and predisposing factors. Clinical Orthopaedics and Related Research. 2008;466(7):1710-5.

[24] Moran E, Masters S, Berendt aR, McLardy-Smith P, Byren I, Atkins BL. Guiding empirical antibiotic therapy in orthopaedics: The microbiology of prosthetic joint infection managed by debridement, irrigation and prosthesis retention. Journal of Infection. 2007;55(1):1-7.

[25] Nimmo GR, Pearson JC, Collignon PJ, Christiansen KJ, Coombs GW, Bell JM, et al. Prevalence of MRSA among Staphylococcus aureus isolated from hospital inpatients, 2005: report from the Australian Group for Antimicrobial Resistance. Communicable Diseases Intelligence. 2007;31(3):288-96.

[26] Peel TN, Cheng AC, Buising KL, Choong PF. The microbiological aetiology, epidemiology and clinical profile of prosthetic joint infections: are current antibiotic prophy-

laxis guidelines effective? Antimicrobial Agents and Chemotherapy. 2012;56(5): 2386-91.

[27] Steckelberg JM, Osmon DR. Prosthetic Joint Infections. In: Waldvogel FA, Bisno AL, editors. Infections Associated with Indwelling Medical Devices. 3rd ed. Washington DC: ASM Press; 2000. p. 173-209.

[28] Weber P, Utzschneider S, Sadoghi P, Andress HJ, Jansson V, Muller PE. Management of the infected shoulder prosthesis: a retrospective analysis and review of the literature. International Orthopaedics. 2011;35(3):365-73.

[29] Piper KE, Jacobson MJ, Cofield RH, Sperling JW, Sanchez-Sotelo J, Osmon DR, et al. Microbiologic diagnosis of prosthetic shoulder infection by use of implant sonication. Journal of Clinical Microbiology. 2009;47(6):1878-84.

[30] Berbari EF, Marculescu C, Sia I, Lahr BD, Hanssen AD, Steckelberg JM, et al. Culture-negative prosthetic joint infection. Clinical Infectious Diseases. 2007;45(9):1113-9.

[31] Murdoch DR, Roberts SA, Fowler VG, Shah MA, Taylor SL, Morris AJ, et al. Infection of orthopedic prostheses after Staphylococcus aureus bacteremia. Clinical Infectious Diseases. 2001;32(4):647-9.

[32] Inman RD, Gallegos KV, Brause BD, Redecha PB, Christian CL. Clinical and microbial features of prosthetic joint infection. American Journal of Medicine. 1984;77(1): 47-53.

[33] Trampuz A, Zimmerli W. Diagnosis and treatment of implant-associated septic arthritis and osteomyelitis. Current Infectious Disease Reports. 2008;10(5):394-403.

[34] Kanafani ZA. Invasive Propionibacterium infections. In: UpToDate, Basow, DS (Ed), UpToDate, Waltham, MA; 2012.

[35] Atkins BL, Athanasou N, Deeks JJ, Crook DWM, Simpson H, Peto TEA, et al. Prospective evaluation of criteria for microbiological diagnosis of prosthetic-joint infection at revision arthroplasty. Journal of Clinical Microbiology 1998;36(10):2932-9.

[36] Parvizi J, Zmistowski B, Berbari E, Bauer T, Springer B, Della Valle C, et al. New definition for periprosthetic joint infection: from the workgroup of the musculoskeletal infection society. Clinical Orthopaedics and Related Research. 2011;469(11):2992-4.

[37] Trampuz A, Piper KE, Jacobson MJ, Hanssen AD, Unni KK, Osmon DR, et al. Sonication of removed hip and knee prostheses for diagnosis of infection. New England Journal of Medicine. 2007;357(7):654-63.

[38] Mirra JM, Amstutz HC, Matos M, Gold R. The pathology of the joint tissues and its clinical relevance in prosthesis failure. Clinical Orthopaedics and Related Research. 1976;117:221-40.

[39] Peel TN, Buising KL, Choong PF. Diagnosis and management of prosthetic joint infection. Current Opinion in Infectious Diseases. 2012;in press.

[40] Marculescu CE, Berbari EF, Hanssen AD, Steckelberg JM, Harmsen SW, Mandrekar JN, et al. Outcome of prosthetic joint infections treated with debridement and retention of components. Clinical Infectious Diseases. 2006;42(4):471-8.

[41] Malekzadeh D, Osmon DR, Lahr BD, Hanssen AD, Berbari EF. Prior use of antimicrobial therapy is a risk factor for culture-negative prosthetic joint infection. Clinical Orthopaedics and Related Research. 2010;468(8):2039-45.

[42] Schafer P, Fink B, Sandow D, Margull A, Berger I, Frommelt L. Prolonged bacterial culture to identify late periprosthetic joint infection: a promising strategy. Clinical Infectious Diseases. 2008;47(11):1403-9.

[43] Brandt CM, Sistrunk WW, Duffy MC, Hanssen aD, Steckelberg JM, Ilstrup DM, et al. Staphylococcus aureus prosthetic joint infection treated with debridement and prosthesis retention. Clinical Infectious Diseases. 1997;24(5):914-9.

[44] Zimmerli W, Frei R, Widmer AF, Rajacic Z. Microbiological tests to predict treatment outcome in experimental device-related infections due to Staphylococcus aureus. Journal of Antimicrobial Chemotherapy. 1994;33:959-67.

[45] Zimmerli W, Widmer AF, Blatter M, Frei R, Ochsner PE. Role of rifampin for treatment of orthopedic implant-related staphylococcal infections: a randomized controlled trial. Journal of the American Medical Association. 1998;279(19):1537-41.

[46] Senneville E, Joulie D, Legout L, Valette M, Dezeque H, Beltrand E, et al. Outcome and predictors of treatment failure in total hip/knee prosthetic joint infections due to Staphylococcus aureus. Clinical Infectious Diseases. 2011;53(4):334-40.

[47] Aboltins CA, Page MA, Buising KL, Jenney AWJ, Daffy JR, Choong PFM. Treatment of staphylococcal prosthetic joint infections with debridement, prosthesis retention and oral rifampicin and fusidic acid. Clinical Microbiology and Infection. 2007;13(6): 586-91.

[48] Forrest GN, Tamura K. Rifampin combination therapy for nonmycobacterial infections. Clinical Microbiology Reviews. 2010;23(1):14-34.

[49] Segreti J, Nelson JA, Trenholme GM. Prolonged suppressive antibiotic therapy for infected orthopedic prostheses. Clinical Infectious Diseases. 1998;27(4):711-3.

[50] Soriano a, Gomez J, Gomez L, Azanza JR, Perez R, Romero F, et al. Efficacy and tolerability of prolonged linezolid therapy in the treatment of orthopedic implant infections. European Journal of Clinical Microbiology and Infectious Diseases. 2007;26(5): 353-6.

[51] Rao N, Regalla DM. Uncertain efficacy of daptomycin for prosthetic joint infections. Clinical Orthopaedics and Related Research. 2006;451:34-7.

[52] John A-K, Baldoni D, Haschke M, Rentsch K, Schaerli P, Zimmerli W, et al. Efficacy of daptomycin in implant-associated infection due to methicillin-resistant Staphylo-

coccus aureus: importance of combination with rifampin. Antimicrobial Agents and Chemotherapy. 2009;53(7):2719-24.

[53] Achermann Y, Clauss M, Derksen L, Raffeiner P, Zellweger C, Eigenmann K, et al. Risk factors for rifampin resistance of staphylococci causing periprosthetic joint infections S 7.4. 29th Annual Meeting of the European Bone and Joint Infection Society; September 2 – 4 Heidelberg, Germany2010.

[54] Deirmengian C, Greenbaum J, Stern J, Braffman M, Lotke PA, Booth RE, Jr., et al. Open debridement of acute gram-positive infections after total knee arthroplasty. Clinical Orthopaedics and Related Research 2003;416(11):129-34.

[55] Meehan AM, Osmon DR, Duffy MC, Hanssen AD, Keating MR. Outcome of penicillin-susceptible streptococcal prosthetic joint infection treated with debridement and retention of the prosthesis. Clinical Infectious Diseases. 2003;36(7):845-9.

[56] Everts RJ, Chambers ST, Murdoch DR, Rothwell AG, McKie J. Successful antimicrobial therapy and implant retention for streptococcal infection of prosthetic joints. ANZ Journal of Surgery 2004;74(4):210-4.

[57] Gaunt PN, Seal DV. Group G streptococcal infection of joints and joint prostheses. Journal of Infection. 1986;13(2):115-23.

[58] Sendi P, Christensson B, Uckay I, Trampuz A, Achermann Y, Boggian K, et al. Group B streptococcus in prosthetic hip and knee joint-associated infections. Journal of Hospital Infection. 2011;79(1):64-9.

[59] Zeller V, Lavigne M, Leclerc P, Lhotellier L, Graff W, Ziza JM, et al. Group B streptococcal prosthetic joint infections: a retrospective study of 30 cases. Presse Medicale. 2009;38(11):1577-84.

[60] Zeller V, Lavigne M, Biau D, Leclerc P, Ziza JM, Mamoudy P, et al. Outcome of group B streptococcal prosthetic hip infections compared to that of other bacterial infections. Joint Bone Spine. 2009;76(5):491-6.

[61] El Helou OC, Berbari EF, Marculescu CE, El Atrouni WI, Razonable RR, Steckelberg JM, et al. Outcome of enterococcal prosthetic joint infection: is combination systemic therapy superior to monotherapy? Clinical Infectious Diseases 2008;47(7):903-9.

[62] Mandell GL, Bennett JE, Dolin R. Principles and Practice of Infectious Diseases. 7th ed. Philadelphia, PA, USA: Churchill Livingstone Elsevier; 2010.

[63] Euba G, Lora-Tamayo J, Murillo O, Pedrero S, Cabo J, Verdaguer R, et al. Pilot study of ampicillin-ceftriaxone combination for treatment of orthopedic infections due to Enterococcus faecalis. Antimicrobial Agents and Chemotherapy. 2009;53(10):4305-10.

[64] Holmberg A, Morgelin M, Rasmussen M. Effectiveness of ciprofloxacin or linezolid in combination with rifampicin against Enterococcus faecalis in biofilms. Journal of Antimicrobial Chemotherapy. 2012;67(2):433-9.

[65] Widmer AF, Wiestner A, Frei R, Zimmerli W. Killing of nongrowing and adherent Escherichia coli determines drug efficacy in device-related infections. Antimicrobial Agents and Chemotherapy. 1991;35(4):741-6.

[66] Hsieh P-H, Lee MS, Hsu K-Y, Chang Y-H, Shih H-N, Ueng SW. Gram-negative prosthetic joint infections: risk factors and outcome of treatment. Clinical Infectious Diseases. 2009;49(7):1036-43.

[67] Aboltins CA, Dowsey MM, Buising KL, Peel TN, Daffy JR, Choong PF, et al. Gram-negative prosthetic joint infection treated with debridement, prosthesis retention and antibiotic regimens including a fluoroquinolone. Clinical Microbiology and Infection. 2011;17(6):862-7.

[68] Legout L, Senneville E, Stern R, Yazdanpanah Y, Savage C, Roussel-Delvalez M, et al. Treatment of bone and joint infections caused by gram-negative bacilli with a cefepime-fluoroquinolone combination. Clinical Microbiology and Infection. 2006;12(10): 1030-3.

[69] McDonald DJ, Fitzgerald RH, Ilstrup DM. Two-stage reconstruction of a total hip arthroplasty because of infection. Journal of Bone and Joint Surgery. 1989;71(6):828-34.

[70] Salvati EA, Chekofsky KM, Brause BD, Wilson PD. Reimplantation in infection. Clinical Orthopaedics and Related Research. 1982;170:62-75.

[71] Tafin UF, Corvec S, Betrisey B, Zimmerli W, Trampuz A. Role of rifampin against Propionibacterium acnes biofilm in vitro and in an experimental foreign-body infection model. Antimicrobial Agents and Chemotherapy 2012;56(4):1885-91.

[72] Bayston R, Nuradeen B, Ashraf W, Freeman BJ. Antibiotics for the eradication of Propionibacterium acnes biofilms in surgical infection. Journal of Antimicrobial Chemotherapy 2007;60(6):1298-301.

[73] Lutz MF, Berthelot P, Fresard A, Cazorla C, Carricajo A, Vautrin AC, et al. Arthroplastic and osteosynthetic infections due to Propionibacterium acnes: a retrospective study of 52 cases, 1995-2002. European Journal of Clinical Microbiology and Infectious Diseases 2005;24(11):739-44.

[74] Zeller V, Ghorbani A, Strady C, Leonard P, Mamoudy P, Desplaces N. Propionibacterium acnes: an agent of prosthetic joint infection and colonization. Journal of Infection. 2007;55(2):119-24.

[75] Azzam K, Parvizi J, Jungkind D, Hanssen A, Fehring T, Springer B, et al. Microbiological, clinical, and surgical features of fungal prosthetic joint infections: a multi-institutional experience. Journal of Bone and Joint Surgery. 2009;91-A Suppl 6:142-9.

[76] Peel T, Daffy J, Thursky K, Stanley P, Buising K. Posaconazole as first line treatment for disseminated zygomycosis. Mycoses. 2008;51(6):542-5.

[77] Johannsson B, Callaghan JJ. Prosthetic hip infection due to Cryptococcus neoformans: case report. Diagnostic Microbiology and Infectious Disease. 2009;64(1):76-9.

[78] Marculescu CE, Berbari EF, Cockerill FR, 3rd, Osmon DR. Fungi, mycobacteria, zoo-
notic and other organisms in prosthetic joint infection. Clinical Orthopaedics and Related Research. 2006;451(10):64-72.

[79] Rex JH, Walsh TJ, Sobel JD, Filler SG, Pappas PG, Dismukes WE, et al. Practice
guidelines for the treatment of candidiasis. Infectious Diseases Society of America.
Clinical Infectious Diseases. 2000;30(4):662-78.

[80] Garcia-Oltra E, Garcia-Ramiro S, Martinez JC, Tibau R, Bori G, Bosch J, et al. Prosthetic joint infection by Candida spp. Rev Esp Quimioter. 2011;24(1):37-41.

[81] Phelan DM, Osmon DR, Keating MR, Hanssen AD. Delayed reimplantation arthroplasty for candidal prosthetic joint infection: a report of 4 cases and review of the literature. Clinical Infectious Diseases. 2002;34(7):930-8.

[82] Uppuluri P, Srinivasan A, Ramasubramanian A, Lopez-Ribot JL. Effects of fluconazole, amphotericin B, and caspofungin on Candida albicans biofilms under conditions of flow and on biofilm dispersion. Antimicrobial Agents and Chemotherapy.
2011;55(7):3591-3.

[83] Bejon P, Berendt A, Atkins BL, Green N, Parry H, Masters S, et al. Two-stage revision
for prosthetic joint infection: predictors of outcome and the role of reimplantation
microbiology. Journal of Antimicrobial Chemotherapy. 2010;65(3):569-75.

Chapter 9

Articulating Spacers in Infection of Total Knee Arthroplasty — State of the Art

Manuel Villanueva-Martínez, Antonio Ríos-Luna,
Francisco Chana-Rodriguez, Jose A. De Pedro and
Antonio Pérez-Caballer

Additional information is available at the end of the chapter

1. Introduction

Infection is one of the most devastating complications of total knee arthroplasty. It is also the leading cause of early revision after knee arthroplasty, ahead of instability and aseptic loosening [1].

Treatment of an infected total knee arthroplasty requires 3 to 6 times more hospital resources than a primary arthroplasty and 2 times more than an aseptic revision [2]. The goal of treatment is to eradicate infection and maintain joint function.

Two-stage exchange remains the treatment of choice in cases of late infection, with good or excellent results in 80% to 100% of cases; nevertheless, it is aggressive, costly, and long. It is also considered the treatment of choice in cases of fungal infection, infection by virulent organisms, inflammatory diseases, immunosuppression, and reinfection after reimplantation.

Compared with direct replacement, 2-stage revision of infected arthroplasty has several disadvantages: longer hospital stay, higher cost, longer surgical time, tissue retraction, instability, and functional limitation between procedures. From a technical standpoint, surgical reimplantation may be hampered by retraction of soft tissue and loss of tissue planes.

Most authors agree that almost all of these problems can be minimized using antibiotic-loaded articulating cement spacers, although 2-stage exchange can be used to eradicate infection both with and without cement spacers.

The most consistent results have been published with 2-stage exchange, regardless of varia-tions in the type of spacer, causal microorganism, or duration of infection. In a systematic review of the literature between 1980 and 2005, Jämsen et al. [3] found 31 original articles describing the results of 154 direct exchanges and 926 2-stage exchanges. Eradication rates were 73%-100% for 1-stage exchange and 82%-100% for 2-stage exchange. Final range of motion and reinfection rates were lower in the series that used antibiotic-loaded articulating spacers. No correlation was observed with the type of spacer or functional outcome between direct revision and 2-stage exchange.

2. Spacer types: Nonarticulating and articulating

The 2-stage exchange protocol was designed by Insall in 1983. Since the first report in 1990, long-term results have shown two-stage exchange to be the treatment of choice for infection after total knee arthroplasty [4]. The outcome of the original procedure was poor to fair in 20% of cases, mainly owing to functional disability and retraction of soft tissue. Atrophy, stiffness, bone loss, and increased extensile exposure were observed at reimplantation.

The use of antibiotic-loaded articulating spacers helped to reduce these complications and improve the possibilities of eradicating infection [5-9]. The choice of spacer depends on many factors, including degree of bone loss, state of the soft tissue, choice of antibiotics, and financial and technical restraints. A benefit that is common to both articulating and nonarticulating antibiotic-loaded spacers is the fact that greater intra-articular levels of antibiotic can be delivered than with parenteral antibiotics [10-11].

The approach aims to be above breakpoint sensitivity (ie, the level of antibiotic that sets the boundary between bacterial susceptibility and the development of resistance) and to eradicate infection.

Nonarticulating spacers enable local administration of a high concentration of antibiotic, improve patient autonomy, facilitate outpatient treatment, and maintain the joint space for future procedures.

Borden and Gearen [5], Booth and Lotke [7], and Cohen et al. [12] reported data for antibiotic-loaded beads and cement spacers, which are molded to adapt to the defect created by removal of the infected prosthesis. Although in some cases these authors made the spacer in 2 semi-blocks, thus forming a partial joint, neither the design of the blocks nor the rehabilitation protocol included controlled mobility. Calton et al. [9] modified this approach, although disadvantages were still observed (eg, bone loss when the spacer sank into the tibia).

Other disadvantages of this system are the minimal range of motion of the joint, which can lead to shortening of the quadriceps, capsule, and ligaments, thus increasing the need for extensile approaches with longer surgical time during reimplantation.

Antibiotic-loaded articulating cement spacers can improve function between operations and facilitate the second stage.

Although this approach remains open to debate, most authors agree that articulating spacers provides better functional results and enable more efficacious eradication of infection than nonarticulating spacers [3], [13-15].

The shape and features of articulating spacers vary considerably, from fully manual spacers made in preformed molds to modular spacers, which include plastic and metal surfaces. Spacers differ in price, complexity, and degree of constraint. The advantages of articulating spacers are as follows: retraction of soft tissue and extensor mechanisms is prevented, high doses of antibiotics can be added in the time between operations, bone mass is preserved better than with nonarticulating spacers[9], [16], the need for expanded approaches at reimplantation is reduced, and the success rate is increased. These approaches also enable greater controlled mobility of the joint and application of a partial support brace, thus facilitating acceptable function between procedures.

3. Historical development of articulating spacers

Use of antibiotic-loaded articulating spacers was first reported by Wilde and Ruth [6] in 1988. This was the first attempt to reduce complications due to functional disability between operations, as observed in the initial work by Windsor and Insall [4].

Preformed articulating systems (PROSTALAC®) first appeared in 1992. Their main advantage was excellent tolerability and function between procedures, thanks to high joint congruence and reduced friction [17]. Their disadvantages include high cost, presence of metal and plastic surfaces that could facilitate bacterial growth, and size limitations. Preformed articulating systems are not widely used because of their price and the theoretical risk that the presence of metal and plastic components facilitates persistence of infection, although this has not been confirmed in clinical practice. Therefore, other factors (eg, aggressiveness of the microorganism, addition of high proportions of cement, and antibiotic treatment) may be more important than the type of spacer used.

Hand-made cement articulating spacers, however, maintain almost all the advantages of preformed spacers, although they also have a series of drawbacks.

Between these extremes, many authors have developed modifications to minimize the disadvantages of hand-made spacers and PROSTALAC® spacers, by adapting them to their technical and economic possibilities. The real impact of the theoretical advantages of the different types of spacer is unknown.

The main forms are as follows:

1. Manual construction of a spacer with cement in the operating room by recreating the normal anatomy of the patient [18], [19] (Figure 1) or more congruent systems (ball and socket) [20] (Figure 2).

2. Construction of customized spacers in the operating room using prefabricated silicone or aluminum molds [21], [22], or using trial components to shape the spacer [23]. Cement

molds can be made during surgery using trial components, and the definitive spacer can be made using these cement molds [24], [25].

3. Prefabricated spacers made of cement only [26].

4. Cement components in combination with modular components made of plastic and metal (PROSTALAC®, DePuy, Warsaw, Indiana) [27], [28].

5. Resterilization of the prosthesis and insertion of a femoral component and a tibial polyethylene insert with cement or a new prosthesis as a spacer (prosthesis-spacer) with high antibiotic loads [29], [30].

6. Combinations of these approaches for moderate or massive defects [31], [32].

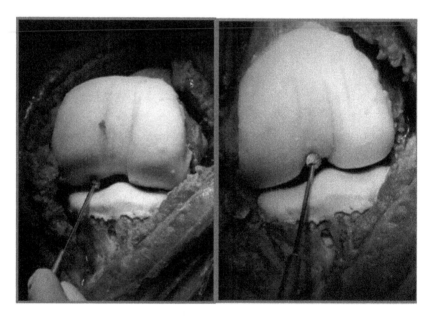

Figure 1. Remodeling prominent areas of a hand-made spacer with a high-speed burr.

Favorable results have been reported with each of these types of spacers. The more rudimentary a spacer is, the lower its congruence and the greater the sensation of popping, giving way, or instability. In contrast, it is cheaper, more widely available, and versatile. The specific advantage of spacers built manually with cement only is that the whole spacer is loaded with antibiotics, and these can be tailored to the causative organism. The spacer does not include plastic, metal, or resterilized parts and can be applied in any operating room with no need for specific instruments. The main disadvantage of cement spacers is the lack of optimal congruence, instability, and the difficulty in modeling, especially with high antibiotic loads (>10%-15%) (Figure3). In addition, cement-on-cement spacers can cause more inflammatory reactions as a result of particle generation; however, this has not been considered a real problem in published series [18], [21], [24].

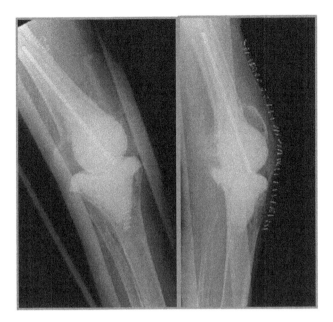

Figure 2. Ball and socket spacer.

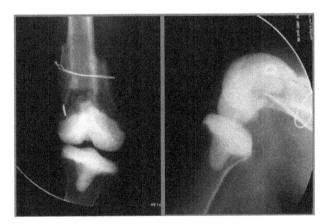

Figure 3. Hand-made spacer for a segmental defect. Excellent range of motion. Due to instability or giving way the patients usually walks with a brace.

Customized spacers constructed completely of cement using prefabricated silicone or aluminum molds are not difficult to shape with greater antibiotic loads.

By contrast, preformed spacers including metal or plastic elements or resterilized prostheses have a limited antibiotic load, which is not tailored to the patient. These spacers involve the insertion of foreign material into a septic environment. In these cases, only the cement fixing the metal components, the prosthesis, or the preformed spacer takes the maximum load of tailored antibiotics.

Also important is the degree of constriction of the spacer. All spacers made intraoperatively with a mold design lack a tibial post and femoral bar; at most, they have a tibial post that gives them some medial-lateral stability. The bar, or lever, which provides anteroposterior stability, is exclusive to PROSTALAC® systems or prosthesis-spacers.

4. Characteristics of antibiotic-loaded spacers

Elution of antibiotics from bone cement depends on several factors: the type of antibiotic, the concentration and combination of antibiotics, the porosity and type of the cement, and the surface of the spacer [33], [34].

4.1. Cement type: Commercially available vs. custom antibiotic-loaded cement

Most commercially available antibiotic-loaded cements, have a low dose of antibiotic, which can act as prophylaxis in patients at risk (ie, double prophylaxis in combination with parenteral antibiotics), or during reimplantation in a 2-stage revision of an infected total knee arthroplasty, but not for the treatment of infection when it is diagnosed[35].

Therefore, surgeons should add antibiotics to the cement to achieve the appropriate doses needed for the treatment of periprosthetic joint infection and to tailor the drug to the causative microorganism.

In comparison with commercial presentations, manually mixed cement releases less antibiotic [33], [34].

Manual mixing of cement and antibiotics increases the porosity of the cement. In theory, this approach weakens the cement, but increases the elution surface, since the antibiotic is released from the surface of the spacer and from cracks in the surface. On the other hand, distribution is not homogeneous (unlike commercially available preloaded cements), thus decreasing the rate of elution from a given surface [36], [37]. One study showed that increasing the surface area of bone cement by 40% yielded a 20% increase in the elution rate of vancomycin [38].

The addition of dextran increases porosity and elution rates. Kuechle et al. [39] noted that when dextran was added at 25%, the release of antibiotics during the first 48 hours was about 4 times greater, and the duration of elution reached 10 days instead of only 6, compared with the routine preparation. The same effect was observed with the addition of lactose and xylitol (or other sugars), which increase the release of daptomycin, vancomycin, and gentamicin [33].

Vacuum mixing decreases the porosity of the cement and thus potentially decreases the elution rate. However, this is not true for all cements, because other factors, such as hydrophilicity or viscosity, may be more important than the area of elution.

In a recent study, Meyer et al. [34] compared the elution of 6 commercially available vacuum-mixed and manually mixed antibiotic-loaded cements. All showed detectable antimicrobial activity during the 5 days of the trial, with peak activity on the first day and levels above breakpoint sensitivity. Levels decreased rapidly thereafter. Cumulative antimicrobial activity during the trial was similar with the manually mixed Cemex Genta and the vacuum-mixed Cobalt G-HV and Palacos RG and higher than that of VersaBond AB, Simplex P with Tobramycin, and SmartSet GMV. The cumulative antimicrobial activity of manually mixed Cemex Genta over 5 days was significantly higher than that of Cobalt G-HV and Palacos RG, which in turn significantly higher cumulative antimicrobial activity than VersaBond AB, Simplex P with Tobramycin, and SmartSet GMV. Vacuum mixing increased the cumulative antimicrobial activity of Cobalt G-HV, Palacos RG, and Simplex P with Tobramycin and decreased the activity of Cemex Genta, SmartSet GMV, and VersaBond AB. The antimicrobial activity was similar for Cobalt G-HV and Palacos RG and significantly higher than that of the other cements. Furthermore, vacuum mixing also increased the number of days of elution above the breakpoint sensitivity necessary to eliminate 99% of methicillin-susceptible *Staphylococcus aureus* (MSSA) and methicillin-resistant *S. aureus* (MRSA) and 85% of coagulase-negative staphylococci (CNS) recorded between 2009 and 2010. For Palacos RG, the number of days of elution increased from 2 days for manually mixed cements to 5 days for vacuum-mixed cements. For Cobalt G-HV, this value increased from 2 to 3 days; for Simplex P with Tobramycin it increased from 1 to 2 days. By contrast, vacuum mixing reduced the number of days' elution above this limit for Cemex Genta from 3 days to 1 day. The authors concluded that vacuum mixing had adverse effects on elution with low-viscosity cement (Cemex Genta), positive effects on elution with high-viscosity cements (Cobalt G-HV and Palacos RG), and unpredictable effects on elution with medium-viscosity cements (Simplex P with Tobramycin, SmartSet GMV, and VersaBond AB). Only manually mixed Cemex Genta and vacuum-mixed Palacos RG eluted antibiotics above breakpoint sensitivity on the third day; the remainder did so only on the first day. Although Cobalt G-HV and Palacos RG have a lower gentamicin load, they have greater antimicrobial activity and elution rates than other cements with a higher antibiotic load.

Other studies confirm differences between cements. Stevens et al. [40] studied the *in vitro* elution of antibiotics from Simplex and Palacos cements and noted that Palacos was a more effective vehicle for local administration [41], [42].

4.2. Choice of antibiotic

Antibiotic-loaded cement spacers release high concentrations of drug and enable higher intra-articular concentrations to be reached than parenteral antibiotics alone, with little effect on serum or urine concentrations and therefore with minimal risk of systemic damage [29], [43], [44]. It is essential to achieve local bactericidal concentrations that make it possible to eradicate infection or prevent colonization of the new implant during the reimplantation phase (the "race for the surface").

The antibiotic used must have 2 fundamental properties:

• Thermostability: Polymerization of the cement is an exothermic reaction. The cement increases in temperature within 10-13 minutes, and this change may alter the properties of the antibiotic.

• Water solubility: The antibiotic is disseminated in the tissues surrounding the infected joint. By maintaining the spacer in the joint for no less than 8 weeks, the antibiotic is released at a constant rate. However, the bactericidal effect is concentrated in the early days. Subsequently, spacers fulfill mainly a mechanical function.

The most frequently used antibiotics are tobramycin, gentamicin, vancomycin, and cephalosporins. Antibiotics can be combined to achieve broad-spectrum coverage, depending on the nature of the causative microorganism. Aminoglycoside in powder is recommended, as it does not weaken the cement; however, it is difficult to obtain in some countries. The surgeon's options are therefore limited when combining antibiotics.

Periprosthetic infections are caused mainly by gram-positive microorganisms (S. aureus and CNS). When the pathogen and its antibiotic sensitivity profile are clearly identified, a single antibiotic should be administered. When the pathogen is unknown, treatment is more difficult, and a combination of antibiotics can improve the chances of eradicating infection. Vancomycin covers MRSA, gentamicin covers Enterobacteriaceae and Pseudomonas aeruginosa, and cefotaxime destroys microorganisms resistant to gentamicin.

In addition to increasing the range of coverage, some combinations of antibiotics have a synergistic effect. Penner et al. [41] observed that the combination of vancomycin and tobramycin acted synergistically, although they discouraged the use of vancomycin in monotherapy. However, other authors have reported excellent results for CNS and MRSA with cement loaded with only 5-7.5% vancomycin (Simplex P, Howmedica, Rutherford, New Jersey, USA: 2-3 g of vancomycin per bag), both in static and in articulating spacers [45].

Synergy between aminoglycosides and vancomycin and, occasionally, a cephalosporin can make it possible to cover a broad spectrum of microorganisms. These antibiotics are usually available in powder form; however, antibiotic-loaded cements are not commercially available. Heraeus are working on a commercial presentation of gentamicin with vancomycin for commercial use in Europe in 2012.

The only commercial presentation with a synergistic effect is Copal, which combines clindamycin and gentamicin. Copal enables increased release of antibiotic and greater ability to inhibit the formation of biofilm than gentamicin alone. Ensing et al. [46] showed that the elution rate of Copal (clindamycin + gentamicin) is much greater than that of other cements, which are also considered excellent [47]. At 7 days, the elution rate was 65% for clindamycin and 41% for gentamicin; for Palacos RG the value for release was 4% for preloaded gentamicin. This increased release of antibiotic resulted in greater and more prolonged inhibition of bacterial growth on agar plates. Gentamicin-susceptible S. aureus strains were "small colony variants" that were resistant to gentamicin in Palacos RG and less so to the gentamicin in Copal. Elution of gentamicin in Palacos RG ceased after 72 hours, in contrast with Copal, which maintained bacterial inhibition during the study period. In addition, unlike Copal, Palacos RG was unable to inhibit bacterial growth of gentamicin-resistant CNS. The addition of clindamycin to gentamicin-loaded cement had an additive effect on the inhibition of biofilm. Conversely, although both cements fulfill ISO norms, the mechanical properties of Palacos RG are superior.

The study by Ensing et al. [46] has several practical implications. Synergy can enable the release of greater amounts of antibiotic, thus making inhibition of bacterial growth more effective and increasing the chances of winning the "race for the surface". By achieving high rates of antibiotic elution, even resistant bacteria can be eradicated when the dose rises sufficiently. Finally, given its worse biomechanical properties, Copal seems ideal for articulating spacers, which are withdrawn after a few weeks, but not as appropriate as Palacos RG for definitive reimplantation once the infection has been cured.

Effective elution from cement has also been observed with quinolones, daptomycin, and linezolid, although these agents are difficult to obtain in powder form or are too expensive [48]. Anguita-Alonso et al. [48] compared quinolones, cefazolin, and linezolid and found linezolid to be the most stable antibiotic after polymerization of PMMA. It achieved high peak concentrations at 7.5% and 15%. All detectable concentrations of linezolid were always above the cutoff sensitivity of *Staphylococcus* spp. (≤ 4 µg/mL).

Daptomycin has also demonstrated the ability to elute in local bactericidal concentrations for *S. aureus* and CNS, with a release profile similar to that of vancomycin [39], [49], [50].

4.3. Fungal infections

In the case of fungal infections, the recommended antibiotic is amphotericin B or fluconazole (Figure 4). 5-Flucytosine is not stable and is therefore not valid for use in cement. Amphotericin can cause nephrotoxicity, hepatotoxicity, chills, nausea, and blood disorders, thus necessitating lower doses and more prolonged treatment. Fortunately, the incidence of fungal infection is low. Most infections are by *Candida* species, of which *C. albicans* accounts for 60%, *C. parapsilosis* 20%, and *C. tropicalis* 20%. More uncommon species include *Coccidioides immitis*, *Sporothrix schenckii*, and *Blastomyces dermatitidis*.

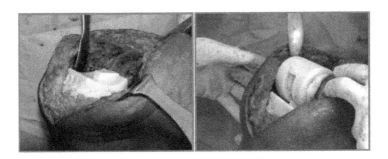

Figure 4. Preformed cement spacer with amphotericin B and fluconazole in a prosthesis with fungal infection.

Immunosuppression, prolonged hospitalization, prolonged intravenous therapy, drug dependence, and inflammatory diseases are risk factors for the development of fungal infections; however, in most published cases the patients did not present these risk factors. A reasonable postulate is that infection is caused by intraoperative inoculation rather than by hematogenous spread. The symptoms are those of a subacute infection, namely, mild to moderate pain or discomfort, effusion, and, occasionally, progressive osteolysis [51]. Published series are very short [52]-[54]. Phelan et al. [55] performed a 2-stage revision procedure with systemic administration of antifungal agents to treat 4 *Candida* infections of total joint arthroplasties. They also identified 6 other cases in the literature that had been treated with the same regimen. In addition to resection arthroplasty, 8 patients received amphotericin B alone or in combination with other antifungal agents, and 1 patient was treated with fluconazole in monotherapy. Eight patients had no recurrence of infection at a mean of 50.7 months after reimplantation.

4.4. Dose of antibiotic

Lewis [33] studied the properties of antibiotic-loaded cements. Elution typically occurs in 3 phases: an exponential phase (during the first 24 hours), a declining phase, and a final low constant elution phase. The exponential phase depends on the diffusion area of the surface of the spacer, although porosity and hydrophilicity of the cement also play a role. Porosity determines the amount of liquid that comes into contact with the surface of the cement, which in turn determines the elution rate of the antibiotic from the surface or from deeper cracks in the cement.

The addition of high doses of antibiotic to the cement is a key element of treatment when attempting to reach maximum intra-articular concentrations in the exponential phase, although some authors have observed persistent effective levels of antibiotics until 4 months after surgery [56].

The antibiotic should not exceed 20% of the total mass of cement. In addition, it should be in powder form, since liquid forms hinder polymerization. No standard ideal dosage of each drug to be mixed with bone cement has been established. Addition of 2 antibiotics to the cement is superior to the addition of 1. The most frequently used doses vary from 2.4 g of tobramycin with 1 g of vancomycin per 40 g of cement to 4 g of vancomycin with 4.6 g of tobramycin per 40 g of cement. These doses have been associated with success rates of above 90% [41], [56].

As the amount of antibiotic powder increases, the strength of the cement decreases. However, antibiotic load seems to be yet another factor within 2-stage exchange, and consistent results have been obtained using unloaded antibiotic spacers or spacers with only minimal loads. Fehring et al. [15] reported efficacious results with 1.2 g of tobramycin per 40 g of bone cement. Mean follow-up was 36 months for patients who received a nonarticulating spacer (88% eradication) and 27 months for patients treated with an articulating spacer (93% eradication).

4.5. Resistance: Mechanical properties of cement

The factors affecting the mechanical properties of the cement are type of cement, proportion and combination of antibiotics, administration in liquid or powder form, and mixing method (manual or vacuum). Cement mixed with cloxacillin, cefazolin, gentamicin, vancomycin, and tobramycin has been shown to maintain good resistance to tension and compression [57], [58].

However, adding liquid antibiotic interferes with early polymerization, leading to a significant deterioration in the properties of the cement, because of the effect of the water and not the properties of the antibiotic itself. For example, addition of liquid gentamicin instead of powder can decrease the resistance of the cement to compression by 49% and the tensile strength by 46%. Tobramycin powder, on the other hand, had not detrimental effects on the spacers [59], [60].

Manually adding antibiotic also weakens the cement. Vacuum-mixed antibiotic-impregnated cement improves its mechanical properties by reducing porosity by up to 20%. It has been estimated that manual mixing causes a 30-40% reduction in resistance and that vacuum mixing can reduce 10-fold the rate of fracture during cyclic loading with spacers [61], [62].

Commercial antibiotic-loaded cements retain their mechanical properties, although the dose may not be sufficient for the treatment of an infection or for the manufacture of spacers, except for some commercial forms, such as Copal.

Duncan [17] reported that manual mixing decreased resistance by 36% with respect to commercially available cement, while the resistance of the latter did not differ from that of nonloaded cement.

Lewis [33] compared several cements and their biomechanical properties after combination with different antibiotics. The composition of the cement was a major factor. The elution rate of vancomycin and tobramycin from Palacos RG is superior to that of Simplex, and the elution rate of Simplex is superior to that of CMW. The combination of antibiotics is also important. Vancomycin combined with tobramycin increases elution with Palacos (the same is true of gentamicin), but with Simplex P, elution of tobramycin decreases, not vice versa. Vacuum mixing also affects elution. CMW variants decrease elution of gentamicin when vacuum-mixed; however, with Palacos the opposite occurs, as confirmed by a recent study [34]. The concentration of vancomycin did not differ significantly depending on whether the cement was mixed manually or by vacuum. These authors also studied the effect of loading and impact cycles, which can lead to minor porosity and cracks in the spacer, thus increasing the elution rate. Among the cements studied, elution only increased with Palamed G, whose porosity is higher. For the remainder, no statistically significant differences were observed between load and lack of impact on the patient.

Also important is the way in which the mixture is made. Hanssen and Spangehl [63] proposed a method for adding high doses of antibiotics to bone cement powder. Polymethylmethacrylate monomer and cement powder must first be mixed to form the liquid cement, and the antibiotic is added afterwards. It is important to leave as many large crystals as possible intact in order to create a more porous mix that increases the elution rate of the antibiotics.

This approach is not applicable when using antibiotic-loaded cement prophylactically, as crystals weaken the cement. Moreover, manual mixing decreases the elution rate in some types of cement. Therefore, commercial forms are preferred.

The method of Frommelt and Kühn [64], namely, fractional addition of antibiotic (now generally recommended), involves the gradual addition of cement and antibiotic powder and mixture of the two until the expected load of antibiotic is complete. The mixture can then be made manually or by vacuum, depending on the type of cement and the availability of vacuum systems. Once mixed, the cement has to be applied in the doughy phase or late phase of polymerization to prevent excessive interdigitation with the bone, thus facilitating extraction during surgery and providing the surgeon with a certain degree of freedom to shape the articular surface of the spacer.

4.6. Safety

As with any treatment, the surgeon must be aware of the possible side effects of the antibiotics used in spacers. Despite the large number of infected arthroplasties treated annually and the widespread use of antibiotic-loaded cement, complications are rare.

Evans [54] used 4 g of vancomycin and 4.6 g of tobramycin in powder per batch of 40 g of polymethylmethacrylate cement in 44 patients with a total of 54 periprosthetic joint infections. Follow-up to a minimum of 2 years showed no renal, vestibular, or auditory effects. Springer et al. [43] studied the systemic safety of cement loaded with high doses of antibiotic over time and reported that an average dose of 10.5 g of vancomycin and 12.5 g of gentamicin was clinically safe, with no signs of acute renal failure or other systemic side effects. In contrast, Van Raaij et al. [65] reported a case of acute renal failure that affected an 83-year-old woman after treatment with 2 g of gentamicin in a 240-g cement block combined with 7 strings of gentamicin-loaded polymethylmethacrylate beads. Serum levels of gentamicin were high, leading to removal of the spacer and eventual recovery of renal function. Ceffa et al. [66] reported 2 cases of mucormycosis after treatment with antibiotic-loaded cement spacers.

The complications reported are rare events in which other factors (eg, blood volume or intravenous antibiotics) could play a role, since the normalization profile of serum antibiotic levels, when using antibiotic-loaded spacers, is exponential and reaches normal values in 24 hours.

5. Results

The use of a polymethylmethacrylate antibiotic-loaded spacer provides not only more effective treatment of periprosthetic infection, with eradication rates ranging from 90% to 100% in the literature, but also improved function, reduced pain, greater patient satisfaction, shorter hospital stay, and lower costs. Few studies analyze developments in the medium-to-long term. Although the results remain more or less stable, up to 30% of patients require revision for loosening, reinfection, or other causes in the medium term [67].

Several studies compare the results of 2-stage exchange with articulating spacers and 28 studies compare the results with a static spacer [3].

Park et al. [68] compared 20 prosthetic knee infections treated with monoblock spacers and 16 treated with articulating spacers. The reinfection rate was 6.3% for the articulating group and 15% for the fixed group. The range of motion with the spacer was 80º and 9º, respectively (final range, 108º and 92º). The clinical and functional score according to the HSS scale was significantly better with the articulating spacer, and the number of extensile exposures was lower. In the static spacer group, 75% of patients (65% of the femurs and 50% of the tibias) had bone loss. This complication was not observed for the articulating spacers.

Meek et al. [27] retrospectively analyzed the results of 2-stage exchange with a PROSTALAC articulating spacer in 47 patients with infected knee prosthesis and a mean follow-up of 41 months. The eradication rate was 96%. The Western Ontario and McMaster Universities Osteoarthritis scale and the Oxford-12 and Short Form-12 scales showed better scores for articulating spacers.

Calton et al. [9] compared the outcomes of patients treated with articulating spacers and patients treated with nonarticulating spacers. Among the 24 patients with a nonarticulating spacer, 60% had an average bone loss of 6.2 mm in the tibia and 12.8 mm in the femur, often with invagination and migration of the spacer and problems of soft tissue retraction. The authors recommended intramedullary extension of the spacer to prevent migration and obtain the appropriate thickness. They also recommended tightening the collateral ligaments to prevent contracture and a block that is sufficiently wide to rest on the cortical rim and prevent migration to cancellous bone. No differences were observed between the groups in eradication rates, time of surgery, or functional outcome.

Fehring et al. [15] studied 25 nonarticulating spacers and 30 articulating spacers and found that articulating spacers facilitated reimplantation and were not associated with bone loss.

Emerson et al. [13] reported that range of motion was greater with articulating knee spacers than with nonarticulating spacers; flexion of the knee averaged 107.8° and 93.7°, respectively, and no evidence of higher complication rates was found.

Therefore, a comprehensive review of the literature provides more arguments for articulating spacers than for static spacers. Articulating spacers seem to be the most widespread form of treatment. The method of making the spacer does not seem to affect eradication rates or functional outcome.

Durbhakula et al. [21] treated 4 patients with antibiotic-loaded articulating spacers made in vacuum-injected silicone molds designed to produce articulating femoral and tibial components. The final average range of motion was 104° and the HSS score was 82. The rate of eradication of infection was 92% after an average of 33 months. A system of this type does not require a metal-polyethylene articulation surface and reduces costs by applying reusable molds that cost about $300 each. The authors reported no problems of dislocation, retraction, bone loss, fracture, or fragmentation of the spacer.

Goldstein et al. [23] formed spacers intraoperatively using cement and test components on aluminum foil to prevent interdigitation. The femoral condyles were molded with the tibial trial implant, and the tibial implant was used to calculate the size and thickness of the cemented tibial component. The authors reported initial success in 5 patients.

MacAvoy and Ries [20] described an inexpensive mold-based method for manufacturing a spherical articulating spacer (ball and socket). They used this method in cases with severe bone deficiency and damage to the ligaments because of its high congruence. The average load was 3.6 g to 4 g of tobramycin + 1 g of vancomycin per bag of Palacos. For an average of 4 cements, this represents a dose of more than 14 g. In 12 patients with severe comorbidities, infection was eradicated in 9 of 13 knees with a mean follow-up of 28 months. All patients could walk with minimal assistance. The average range of motion of the knee with the spacer was 79°, which increased to 98° at the end of treatment. The authors rarely used hinge models, despite serious injury to the ligaments and bone loss.

Using cement spacer molds created intraoperatively with Palacos RG loaded with 0.5 g of gentamicin plus 3 g of vancomycin, Shen et al. [25] obtained 10 reimplantations in 17 cases followed for 30 months. In 5 cases, the spacer was the definitive treatment, in 1 case the joint merged, and 1 patient required amputation. The average range of motion with the spacer was 82° (97° after reimplantation).

Excellent results have been reported with the Hoffman prosthesis-spacer system. Anderson et al. [30] reported a range of motion of 2° to 115°; Huang et al. [69] reported 97.6°, which was smaller than in previous publications (104º to 115º). As for eradication with this type of spacer, reinfection rates are variable: 4% according to Anderson et al. [30] (25 knees), 0%-12% according to Hofmann et al. [29] (22 and 50 patients; Simplex cement with 4.8 g of vancomycin per bag), 9% according to Emerson et al. [13] (22 patients), and 2% according to Cuckler [70] (44 patients).

Ha [24] reported motion ranging from 2° to 104° with manually modeled cement spacers. The study included 12 cases treated with spacers made using the double mold (a cement negative is made with trial components and the definitive spacer is modeled on the negative) and using doses of 4.8 g of tobramycin and 4 g of vancomycin per cement bag. The antibiotic load accounted for 20% of the cement-antibiotic composite.

In addition to the type of spacer, range of motion is influenced by preoperative mobility, the state of the soft tissues, surgical technique, implant selection, early rehabilitation, and patient cooperation. Our group [18] found the range of motion to be 107° after reimplantation using manual spacers and 7.5% antibiotic load.

Soft tissue damage, severe bone loss or general health status, appear to be more important than the treatment method, and the results of 2-stage exchange, which are generally excellent, are much worse in patients with a less favorable health status.

Macmull et al. [71] published 19 cases with the SMILES spacer, which was based on an antibiotic-loaded hinge coated with antibiotic-loaded cement (Palacos RG, Heraeus Medical GmbH, Wehrheim, Germany). The spacer was used in the early stages of chronic infection associated with severe bone loss on revision arthroplasty in 11 cases (58%), tumor endoprostheses in 4 (21%), primary arthroplasty in 2 (11%), and infection on fracture or osteotomy in 2. The eradication rate at 38 months was 63% (12 cases), Four patients (21%) suffered reinfection and 2 were amputees. Jeys et al. [72] reported an eradication rate of 72% in primary infection of massive tumor prosthesis with a 2-stage protocol.

Reinfection after reimplantation has not been adequately studied in the literature, although the high percentage of rescue treatments indicates that reinfection has its own prognostic implications. Therefore, it could be classified as a separate type of infection and independently studied in the future.

Hanssen et al. [73] published a series of 24 reinfections after infected total knee prosthesis. The infection was eradicated in only 1 case. Another patient received suppressive therapy after a new reimplantation, and the rest underwent arthrodesis.

Hart and Jones [74] reported 6 cases of reinfection following 2-stage revision. The infection was eradicated in 2 cases (with another 2-stage revision), 2 patients had bone fusions, and 2 had suppressive treatments.

6. Conclusions

1. Two-stage exchange is considered the treatment of choice in the following circumstances: late infection, unidentified causal microorganisms, fungal infections, infections by virulent organisms, underlying inflammatory diseases, immunosuppression, and reinfection after reimplantation.

2. Articulating spacers can minimize complications between procedures, thus enhancing patient autonomy and mobility, preventing retraction of the soft tissues, and facilitating reimplantation.

3. In addition, articulating spacers seem to improve eradication rates and functional outcomes and reduce complications.

4. The way the spacer is constructed does not seem to affect eradication rates and functional outcome. The surgeon's choice of spacer will depend on technical and financial restraints. Despite their advantages and disadvantages, all types of spacer have demonstrated consistent and reproducible results.

5. Not all cements are equally suitable for the prevention and treatment of infection.

6. The antibiotic should be added as powder to avoid weakening the cement. Appropriate use of synergies increases the spectrum of coverage and elution rate of certain antibiotics.

7. Once fractionated addition is complete, vacuum mixing increases the elution of the antibiotic from the spacer when high-viscosity cements are used. Manual mixing is preferred when low-viscosity cements are used.

Author details

Manuel Villanueva-Martínez[1*], Antonio Ríos-Luna[2], Francisco Chana-Rodriguez[1], Jose A. De Pedro[3] and Antonio Pérez-Caballer[4]

*Address all correspondence to: mvillanuevam@yahoo.com

1 Hospital General Universitario Gregorio Marañón, Universidad Complutense de Madrid, Madrid, Spain

2 Orthoindal Center, El Ejido, Almería University, Almería, Spain

3 Hospital Universitario Salamanca, Salamanca University, Spain

4 Hospital Infanta Elena, Francisco de Vitoria University, Madrid, Spain

References

[1] Sharkey, P. F, Hozack, W. J, Rothman, R. H, Shastri, S, & Jacoby, S. M. Why Are Total Knee Arthroplasties Failing Today?. Clin Orthop (2002). , 404, 7-13.

[2] Iorio, R, Healy, W. L, & Richards, J. A. Comparison of the hospital cost of primary and revision total knee arthroplasty after cost containment. Orthopedics (1999). , 22, 195-199.

[3] Jämsen, E, Stogiannidis, I, Malmivaara, A, Pajamäki, J, Puolakka, T, & Konttinen, Y. T. Outcome of prosthesis exchange for infected knee arthroplasty: the effect of treatment approach. A systematic review of the literature. Acta Orthopaedica (2009). , 80, 67-77.

[4] Windsor, R. E, Insall, J. N, Urs, W. K, Miller, D. V, & Brause, B. D. Two-stage reimplantation for the salvage of total knee arthroplasty complicated by infection: further follow-up and refinement of indications. J Bone Joint Surg Am (1990). A.: 272-8., 72.

[5] Borden, L. S. Gearen PF: Infected total knee arthroplasty: A protocol for management. J Arthroplasty (1987). , 2, 27-36.

[6] Wilde, A. H, & Ruth, J. T. Two stage reimplantation in infected total knee arthroplasty. Clin Orthop (1988). , 23-35.

[7] Booth, R. E, & Lotke, P. A. The results of spacer block technique in revision of infected total knee arthroplasty. Clin Orthop (1989).

[8] Hoffman, A. A, Kane, K. R, Tkach, T. K, Plaster, R. L, & Camargo, M. P. Treatment of infected total knee replacement arthroplasty using an articulating spacer. Clin Orthop (1995). , 321, 44-54.

[9]   Calton, T. F, Fehring, T. K, & Griffin, W. L. Bone loss associated with the use of spacer blocks in infected total knee arthroplasty. Clin Orthop (1997). , 345, 148-54.

[10] Jiranek, W. A, Arlen, D, Hanssen, A. D, & Greenwald, A. S. Antibiotic-loaded bone cement for infection prophylaxis in total joint replacement. J Bone Joint Surg Am. (2006). , 88, 2487-2500.

[11] Alt, V, Bechert, T, & Steinrücke, P. In vitro testing of antimicrobial activity of bone cement. Antimicrob Agents Chemother (2004). , 48, 4084-8.

[12] Cohen, J. C, Hozack, W. J, Cucker, J. M, & Booth, R. E. Two stage reimplantation of septic total knee arthroplasty: report of three cases using an antibiotic PMMA spacer block. J Arthroplasty (1988). , 3, 369-77.

[13] Emerson Jr RHMuncie M, Tarbox TR, Higgins LL. Comparison of a static with a mobile spacer in total knee infection. Clin Orthop (2002). , 404, 132-8.

[14] Cui, Q, Mihalko, W. M, Shields, J. S, Ries, M, & Saleh, K. J. Antibiotic-impregnated cement spacers for the treatment of infection associated with total hip or knee arthro-plasty. J Bone Joint Surg Am (2007). , 89, 871-82.

[15] Fehring, T. K, Odum, S, Calton, T. F, & Mason, J. B. Articulating versus static spacers in revision total knee arthroplasty for sepsis. The Ranawat Award. Clin Orthop (2000). , 380, 9-16.

[16] Chiang, E. R, Su, Y. P, Chen, T. H, Chiu, F. Y, & Chen, W. M. Comparison of articulating and static spacers regarding infection with resistant organisms in total knee arthro-plasty. Acta Orthopaedica (2011). , 82, 460-464.

[17] Duncan, C. P, Beauchamp, C. P, & Masri, B. The antibiotic loaded joint replacement system: A novel approach to the management of the infected knee replacement. J Bone Joint Surg Br (1992). suppl III): 296

[18] Villanueva-martínez, M, Ríos-luna, A, Pereiro, J, & Fahandez-saddi, H. Hand-made articulating spacers in two-stage revision for infected total knee arthroplasty: good outcome in 30 patients. Acta Orthop Scand (2008). , 79, 674-82.

[19] Mcpherson, E. J, Lewonowski, K, & Dorr, L. D. Techniques in arthroplasty. Use of an articulated PMMA spacer in the infected total knee arthroplasty. J Arthroplasty (1995). , 10, 87-89.

[20] MacAvoy MCRies MD. The ball and socket articulating spacer for infected total knee arthroplasty. J Arthroplasty (2005). , 20, 757-62.

[21] Durbhakula, S. M, Czajka, J, Fuchs, M. D, & Uhl, R. L. Antibiotic-loaded articulating cement spacer in the 2-stage exchange of infected total knee arthroplasty. J Arthroplasty (2004). , 19, 768-74.

[22] Hsu, Y. C, Cheng, H. C, & Ng, T. P. Antibiotic-loaded cement articulating spacer for 2-stage reimplantation in infected total knee arthroplasty: a simple and economic method. J Arthroplasty (2007). , 22, 1060-6.

[23] Goldstein, W. M, Kopplin, M, Wall, R, & Berland, K. Temporary articulating methyl-methacrylate antibiotic spacer (TAMMAS): a new method of intraoperative manufac-turing of a custom articulating spacer. J Bone Joint Surg. (2001). S, 2, 92-97.

[24] Ha, C. W. A technique for intraoperative construction of antibiotic spacers. Clin Orthop (2006). , 445, 204-9.

[25] Shen, H, Zhang, X, Jiang, Y, Wang, Q, & Chen, Y. Qi Wang Q, Shao J. Intraoperatively-made cement-on-cement antibiotic-loaded articulating spacer for infected total knee arthroplasty. The Knee (2010). , 17(2010), 407-411.

[26] Pitto, R. P, Castelli, C. C, Ferrari, R, & Munro, J. Pre-formed articulating knee spacer in two-stage revision for the infected total knee arthroplasty. Int Orthop (2005). , 29, 305-8.

[27] Meek, R. M, Masri, B. A, Dunlop, D, Garbuz, D. S, Greidanus, N. V, Mcgraw, R, & Duncan, C. P. Patient satisfaction and functional status after treatment of infection at the site of a total knee arthroplasty with use of the PROSTALAC articulating spacer. J Bone Joint Surg Am (2003). , 85, 1888-92.

[28] Haddad, F. S, Masri, B. A, Campbell, D, Mcgraw, R. W, Beauchamp, C. P, & Duncan, C. P. The PROSTALAC functional spacer in two-stage revision for infected knee replacements: prosthesis of antibiotic-loaded acrylic cement. J Bone Joint Surg Br (2000). , 82, 807-12.

[29] Hofmann, A. A, Goldberg, T, Tanner, A, & Kurtin, S. M. Treatment of infected total knee arthroplasty using an articulating spacer: 2- to 12-year experience. Clin Orthop (2005). , 430, 125-31.

[30] Anderson, J. A, Sculco, P. K, Heitkemper, S, Mayman, D. J, Bostrom, M. P, & Sculco, T. P. An articulating spacer to treat and mobilize patients with infected total knee arthroplasty. J Arthroplasty (2009). , 24, 631-5.

[31] Incavo, S. J, Russell, R. D, Mathis, K. B, & Adams, H. Initial Results of Managing Severe Bone Loss in Infected Total Joint Arthroplasty Using Customized Articulating Spacers. J Arthroplasty. (2009). , 24, 607-13.

[32] Macmull, S, Bartlett, M. J, Blunn, G. W, Pollock, R. C, Carrington, R. W, Skinner, J. A, Cannon, S. R, & Briggs, T. W. Custom-made hinged spacers in revision knee surgery for patients with infection, bone loss and instability. The Knee (2010). , 17, 403-406.

[33] Lewis, G. Review Properties of Antibiotic-Loaded Acrylic Bone Cements for Use in Cemented Arthroplasties: A State-of-the-Art Review. J Biomed Mater Res Part B: Appl Biomater (2009). B: , 558-574.

[34] Meyer, J, Piller, G, Spiegel, C. A, Hetzel, S, & Squire, M. Vacuum-Mixing Significantly Changes Antibiotic Elution Characteristics of Commercially Available Antibiotic-Impregnated Bone Cements. J Bone Joint Surg Am (2011). , 93, 2049-56.

[35] Dunne, N, Hill, J, Mcafee, P, Todd, K, Kirkpatrick, R, Tunney, M, & Patrick, S. In vitro study of the efficacy of acrylic bone cement loaded with supplementary amounts of gentamicin. Effect on mechanical properties, antibiotic release, and biofilm formation. Acta Orthopaedica (2007). , 78(6), 774-785.

[36] Nelson, C. L, Griffin, F. M, Harrison, B. H, & Cooper, R. E. In vitro elution characteristics of commercially and noncommercially prepared antibiotic PMMA beads. Clin Orthop Relat Res. (1992). , 284, 303-9.

[37] Kuehn, K. D, Ege, W, & Gopp, U. Acrylic bone cements: composition and properties. Orthop Clin North Am. (2005). , 36, 17-28.

[38] Greene, N, Holtom, P. D, Warren, C. A, Ressler, R. L, Shepherd, L, Mcpherson, E. J, & Patzakis, M. J. In vitro elution of tobramycin and vancomycin polymethylmethacrylate beads and spacers from Simplex and Palacos. Am J Orthop (1998). , 27, 201-205.

[39] Kuechle, D. K, Landon, G. C, Musher, D. M, & Noble, P. C. Elution of vancomycin, daptomycin, and amikacin from acrylic bone cement. Clin Orthop Relat Res (1991). , 264, 302-8.

[40] Stevens, C. M, Tetsworth, K. D, Calhoun, J. H, & Mader, J. T. An articulated antibiotic spacer used for infected total knee arthroplasty: a comparative in vitro elution study of Simplex and Palacos bone cements. Journal of Orthopaedic Researh (2005). , 23, 27-33.

[41] Penner, M. J, Masri, B. A, & Duncan, C. P. Elution characteristics of vancomycin and tobramycin combined in acrylic bone-cement. J Arthroplasty. (1996). , 11, 939-44.

[42] Greene, N, Holtom, P. D, Warren, C. A, Ressler, R. L, Shepherd, L, Mcpherson, E. J, & Patzakis, M. J. In vitro elution of tobramycin and vancomycin polymethylmethacrylate beads and spacers from Simplex and Palacos. Am J Orthop. (1998). , 27, 201-5.

[43] Springer, B. D, Lee, G. C, Osmon, D, Haidukewych, G. J, Hanssen, A. D, & Jacofsky, D. J. Systemic safety of high-dose antibiotic-loaded cement spacers after resection of an infected total knee arthroplasty. Clin Orthop Relat Res (2004). , 427, 47-51.

[44] Hanssen, A. D, & Spangehl, M. J. Practical applications of antibiotic-loaded bone cement for treatment of infected joint replacements. Clin Orthop Relat Res (2004). , 427, 79-85.

[45] Chiang, E. R, Su, Y. P, Chen, T. H, Chiu, F. Y, & Chen, W. M. Comparison of articulating and static spacers regarding infection with resistant organisms in total knee arthroplasty. Acta Orthopaedica (2011). , 82(4), 460-464.

[46] Ensing, G. T, Van Horn, J. R, Van Der Mei, H. C, Busscher, H. J, & Neut, D. Copal Bone Cement Is More Effective in Preventing Biofilm Formation than Palacos R-G. Clin Orthop Relat Res (2008). , 466, 1492-1498.

[47] Neut, D, De Groot, E. P, Kowalski, R. S, Van Horn, J. R, Van Der Mei, H. C, & Busscher, H. J. Gentamicin-loaded bone cement with clindamycin or fusidic acid added: biofilm formation and antibiotic release. J Biomed Mater Res (2005). , 165-170.

[48] Anguita-alonso, P, Rouse, M. S, Piper, K. E, Jacofsky, D. J, Osmon, D. R, & Patel, R. Comparative study of antimicrobial release kinetics from polymethylmethacrylate. Clin Orthop Relat Res (2006). , 445, 239-244.

[49] Webb, N. D, Mccanless, J. D, Courtney, H. S, Bumgardner, J. D, & Haggard, W. O. Daptomycin Eluted From Calcium Sulfate Appears Effective Against Staphylococcus. Clin Orthop Relat Res. (2008). , 466(6), 1383-1387.

[50] Hall, E. W, Rouse, M. S, Jacofsky, D. J, Osmon, D. R, Hanssen, A. D, Steckelberg, J. M, & Patel, R. Release of daptomycin from polymethylmethacrylate beads in a continuous flow chamber. Diagnostic Microbiology and Infectious Disease (2004). , 50, 261-265.

[51] Wyman, J, Mcgough, R, & Limbird, R. Fungal infection of a total knee prosthesis: Successful treatment using articulating cement spacers and staged reimplantation. Orthopedics (2002). , 25, 1391-4.

[52] Baumann, P. A, Cunningham, B, Patel, N. S, & Finn, H. A. Aspergillus fumigatus infection in a mega prosthetic total knee arthroplasty: salvage by staged reimplantation with 5-year follow-up. J Arthroplasty (2001). , 16, 498-503.

[53] Langer, P, Kassim, R. A, Macari, G. S, & Saleh, K. J. Aspergillus infection after total knee arthroplasty. Am J Orthop (2003). , 32, 402-4.

[54] Evans, R. P. Successful treatment of TH and TK infection with articulating antibiotic components. A modified treatment method. Clin Orthop Relat Research. (2004). , 427, 37-46.

[55] Phelan, D. M, Osmon, D. R, Keating, M. R, & Hanssen, A. D. Delayed reimplantation arthroplasty for candidal prosthetic joint infection: a report of 4 cases and review of the literature. Clin Infect Dis (2002). , 34, 930-8.

[56] Masri, B. A, Duncan, C. P, & Beauchamp, C. P. Long-term elution of antibiotics from bone-cement: an in vivo study using the prosthesis of antibiotic-loaded acrylic cement (PROSTALAC) system. J Arthroplasty (1998). , 13, 331-8.

[57] Armstrong, M. S, Spencer, R. F, Cunningham, J. L, Gheduzzi, S, Miles, A. W, & Learmonth, I. D. Mechanical characteristics of antibiotic-laden bone cement. Acta Orthop Scand (2002). , 73, 688-90.

[58] Klekamp, J, Dawson, J. M, Haas, D. W, Deboer, D, & Christie, M. The use of vancomycin and tobramycin in acrylic bone cement: biomechanical effects and elution kinetics for use in joint arthroplasty. J Arthroplasty (1999). , 14, 339-46.

[59] Seldes, R. M, Winiarsky, R, Jordan, L. C, Baldini, T, Brause, B, Zodda, F, & Sculco, T. P. Liquid gentamicin in bone cement: a laboratory study of a potentially more cost-effective cement spacer. J Bone Joint Surg Am (2005). , 87, 268-72.

[60] Deluise, M, & Scott, C. P. Addition of hand-blended generic tobramycin in bone cement: effect on mechanical strength. Orthopedics (2004). , 27, 1289-91.

[61] Kuehn, K. D, Ege, W, & Gopp, U. Acrylic bone cements: mechanical and physical properties. Orthop Clin North Am (2005). , 36, 29-39.

[62] Kuehn, K. D, Ege, W, & Gopp, U. Acrylic bone cements: composition and properties. Orthop Clin North Am (2005). , 36, 17-28.

[63] Hanssen, A. D, & Spangehl, M. J. Treatment of the infected hip replacement. Clin Orthop Relat Res (2004). , 420, 63-71.

[64] Frommelt, L, & Kühn, K. D. Antibiotic-loaded cement. In: Breusch SJ, Malchau M. The well-cemented total hip arthroplasty. Heidelberg: Springer, (2005). , 86-92.

[65] Van Raaij, T. M, Visser, L. E, Vulto, A. G, & Verhaar, J. A. Acute renal failure after local gentamicin treatment in an infected total knee arthroplasty. J Arthroplasty (2002). , 17, 948-50.

[66] Ceffa, R, Andreoni, S, Borre, S, Ghisellini, F, Fornara, P, Brugo, G, & Ritter, M. A. Mucoraceae infections of antibiotic-loaded cement spacers in the treatment of bacterial infections caused by knee arthroplasty. J Arthroplasty (2002). , 17, 235-8.

[67] Haleem, A. A, Berry, D. J, & Hanssen, A. D. Mid-Term to Long-Term Followup of Two-stage Reimplantation for Infected Total Knee Arthroplasty. Clin Orthop Relat Research (2004). , 428, 35-39.

[68] Park, S. J, Song, E. K, Seon, J. K, Yoon, T. R, & Park, Y. H. Comparison of static and mobile antibiotic-impregnated cement spacers for the treatment of infected total knee arthroplasty. International Orthopaedics (SICOT) (2010). , 34, 1181-1186.

[69] Huang, H, Su, J, & Chen, S. The results of articulating spacer technique for infected total knee arthroplasty. J Arthroplasty (2006). , 21, 1163-8.

[70] Cuckler, J. M. The infected total knee. Management options. J Arthroplasty (2005). S , 2, 33-6.

[71] Macmull, S, Bartlett, W, Miles, W, Blunn, J, Pollock, G. W, Carrington, R. C, Skinner, R. W, Cannon, J. A, Briggs, S. R, & Custom-made, T. W. hinged spacers in revision knee surgery for patients with infection, bone loss and instability. The Knee (2010). , 17, 403-406.

5

[72] Jeys, J L. M, Grimer, S. R, & Tillman, R. M. Periprosthetic infection in patients treated for an orthopaedic oncological condition. Bone Jt Surg Am (2005). , 87, 842-9.

[73] Hanssen, A. D, Trousdale, R. T, & Osmon, D. R. Patient outcome with reinfection following reimplantation for the infected total knee arthroplasty. Clin Orth Relat Res (1995). , 321, 55-67.

[74] Hart, W. J, & Jones, R. S. Two-stage revision of infected total knee replacements using articular cement spacers and short-term antibiotic therapy. J Bone J Surg Br (2006). , 88, 1011-5.

Chapter 10

The Role of Knee Arthrodesis After TKA Infection

Pablo Renovell, Antonio Silvestre and
Oscar Vaamonde

Additional information is available at the end of the chapter

1. Introduction

Infection after total knee arthroplasty (TKA) is a devastating complication posing substantial clinical and financial burden, which incidence is increasing in line with the rise of the number of TKAs performed worldwide. The incidence of this complication rates from 1% in primary TKAs to 5.8% after TKAs revision in long series [1]. The lowest reinfection rate after a prior reimplantation for septic TKA has been reported near 30% [2].

The goals in the treatment of chronic infected TKA are control of the disease and restoring knee function. Alternative techniques in the management of reinfected knee prosthesis are another two-stage prosthesis reimplantation, arthrodesis, resection arthroplasty, and supra-condylar amputation [3]. Although two-stage surgery is generally believed as the most successful decision, chronic infection forces surgeons to look for other alternatives.

Recurring infection at the site of a total knee arthroplasty should be treated by knee arthrodesis unless control of the disease and good functional recover could be possible [4]. Arthrodesis of the knee can provide a stable painless joint for an independent lifestyle that would not be possible after a failed total knee replacement. Whereas reimplantation of a TKA shows better limb function, arthrodesis achieves better pain relief, not finding significant differences in knee scores between the two procedures (Oxford knee score) [5, 6]. Knee arthrodesis can be achieved with a cemented or uncemented intramedullary nail, inserted from great trochanter or through the knee, with two plates applied in two planes or using an external fixator to produce a joint fusion [4]. Intramedullary nails provide greater stability, avoid pin-track infection, allow faster weight bearing and generally are better accepted by the patients than external fixators [7]. Illizarov method is more desirable when soft tissues conditions are poor or after failing of intramedullary nail [8, 9].

There are few and short series of cemented modular nail for knee arthrodesis after TKA infection in literature [10, 11]. The purpose of this study is to report the role of knee arthrodesis after chronic infection of knee prostheses and show our results with the use of a modular cemented nail inserted through the knee.

2. Material and methods

We review retrospectively twenty-one patients who have undergone knee arthrodesis with a cemented modular nail for chronic infection of knee prosthesis, from January 2003 until January 2011 in our Department. Three senior surgeons performed all procedures.

Endo-Model® Knee Fusion Nail (Newsplint, UK/Waldemar Link®, Gmbh & Co. KG, Hamburg, Germany) was used in all cases. Twelve of those cases received previous surgery in our Hospital (a reference institution for knee reconstruction) but the other nine cases came from others Hospitals. The decision to undertake knee fusion was arranged after analyzing the different options with the patient.

The first surgical stage was exhaustive debridement and placement of a double antibiotic-loaded (clindamycin and gentamicin) bone cement as a static spacer (Rofabacin® Revision, Biomet®). Systemic antibiotics according to the culture results were given to the patients for at least six weeks. When the patient was recovered from the first-stage surgery, no signs of infection were observed and values of inflammatory markers (PCR and ESR) were decreased, the cemented modular nail was inserted through the knee after reaming tibial and femoral canals. Tibial and femur implants are cemented with antibiotic loaded cement. Nineteen cases were performed according to this two-stage procedure, but two cases were done in just one-stage.

Hospital records and serial radiographies of all patients were reviewed to evaluate patient status and outcomes. We have excluded a patient lost on follow-up.

Number of previous surgeries per patient, comorbidities and microorganisms responsible for the infection were recorded.

In order to assess functional outcome, the Oxford Knee Score (OKS) [12] was checked before removal of the implants and at final follow-up. Successful outcome was defined as not or slight pain on the operated limb and able to walk with or without aids at the time of the last follow-up.

3. Results

Twenty-one patients were treated with cemented modular nail for knee arthrodesis from 2003 to 2011 for chronic infection of the prostheses (Figure 1.). One patient was lost during follow-up and was excluded from this series. Mean follow-up of patients was 3.2 years (range, six months to eight years).

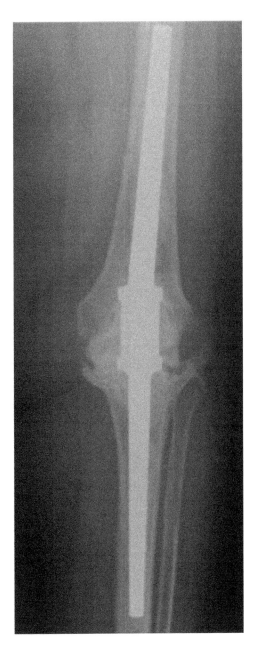

Figure 1. Cemented modular nail for knee arthrodesis.

Twenty patients were fully recorded. The series includes eleven women and nine men with a mean age of seventy-six years (range 68-86 years) at the time of arthrodesis. Time since primary knee arthroplasty until knee arthrodesis, ranged from eight months to nine years (mean 4.4 years). The number of procedures carried out before definitive arthrodesis ranged from 2 to 7 (mean 3.3 surgeries).

Most frequent comorbidities were hypertension (65%), obesity [BMI>30kg/m²] (45%) and Diabetes Mellitus (40%). Demographics of the patients are shown in Table 1.

Number of patients fully recorded	20
Age	76.8±10.2
Sex (M/F)	11/9
Side (R/L)	12/8
Body mass index (Kg/m²)	29.8±1.4
Comorbidities	
HTA	13 (65%)
Obesity	9 (45%)
DM	8 (40%)
Mean nº of knee prior surgeries	3.3(2-7)
Preoperative OKS	17.1 (9-32)

Table 1. Demographics of the study population

Intraoperative cultures were positive on 19 cases (95%). In eight of the cases (40%) only one bacteria could be checked, but on the other hand two or more microorganisms yielded on cultures in eleven cases (55%). The predominant microorganisms were *staphylococcus epidermidis* in 11 cases (55%) and *staphylococcus aureus* in 7 cases (35%), 10 of which (8 *s. epidermidis* and 2 *s. aureus*) were *methicillin-resistant staphylococcus (MRS)*, so we can conclude that 50% of fused knees were positive to MRS. Other microorganism included in this series was *Escherichia coli* in 4 cases (20%).

Fifteen patients (75%) healed without problems and they did not need more surgeries, four (20%) showed inadequate control of infection so required new performances (one case one-stage debridement, two arthrodesis with external fixators and one case supracondylar amputation), and two cases (10%) suffered a tibial shaft fracture below the tip of the nail. One of the fractures was resolved changing the nail for a longer one (Figure 2), and the other was treated with immobilization. Two of the four cases (50%) with persistence of of infection were operated in one-stage surgery.

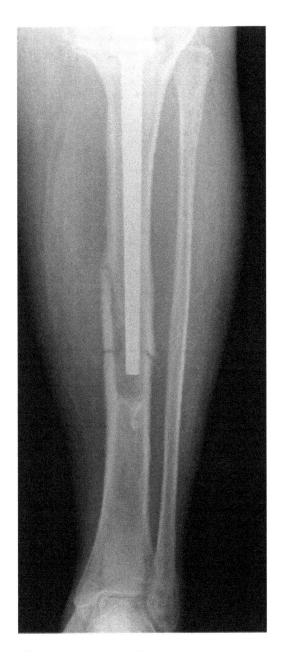

Figure 2. Tibia fracture and bone loosening below the nail.

The mean Oxford knee score improved from 17.1 points (range, 9 to 32 points) before removal of the prosthesis, to 27.4 points (range, 6 to 41 points) postoperatively. Successful outcome was 95% at the time of the last follow-up. Results of the series are shown in Table 2.

Number of cases infected by MRS	10 (50%)
Patients healed without problems	15 (75%)
Causes of reoperations	
Persistent infection	4 (20%)
Fracture on tibia below the nail (and bone loosening)	1 (5%)
Reoperations	
Arthrodesis with external fixator 2	
One-stage debridement	1
Supracondylar amputation	1
Change for a longer nail	1
Postoperative OKS	27.4 (6-41)

Table 2. Results of knee arthrodesis with cemented modular nail

4. Discussion

The reason to turn a TKA into arthrodesis due to a chronic infection is not clear nowadays, and the decision-making process is sometimes difficult. When a second infection happens, the number of surgeries performed in the knee reaches until 9.3 of average [1], so this detail must be always present on surgeon's mind when re-infection occurs. Infection of primary TKA has been related with hyperglycaemia, prolonged operative time, obesity, rheumatoid arthritis and others [1], however in TKA reinfection, the main factors related to this condition are previous infection with tough microorganisms, poor soft tissue coverage and number of previous surgeries [2].

Although surgeon might consider joint fusion as a poor result, comparing to other choices, knee with a fusion is more efficient and functional [13]. Supracondylar amputation as a consequence of a failed total knee revision arthroplasty is a salvage procedure in front of a severe infection, uncontrolled pain or massive bone loss. This radical surgery should not be related knee prosthesis complications but to peripheral vascular disease or recurrence of a malignant tumor [14]. Functional outcome after supracondylar amputation carried out ought to an infected total knee replacement is poor. Patients with a supracondylar amputation after chronic infection of prosthesis show low functional status. Only 50% of these patients are able to walk after the surgery [15]. The awful OKS of our amputated patients (6 points), confirms this fact.

The alternative of resection arthroplasty in case of recalcitrant TKA infection is only an option when the patient previously was not able to walk, due to a medical infirmity or other limb pathology. Results on pain and functional scores are always lower than two-stage reimplatation or arthrodesis [16].

Clinical outcomes of revision TKA after aseptic loosening are better than knee prosthesis revision after chronic infection [17]. Wang et al [5] asserted, comparing clinical outcomes of the different alternatives in the treatment of infected TKA, that Oxford Knee Score after revision TKA is similar to knee arthrodesis. He reported just about mild-to-moderate knee pain on almost 50% of the reimplanted TKAs. Knee arthrodesis shows better pain relief but worse function than revision TKA, whereas reimplanted TKA reveals better function and worse pain relief than knee fusion. Anyway, knee arthrodesis allows the patient an independent lifestyle with few complications [18]. And it is important to keep in mind that re-infection rate after TKA revision is 68.6%, lessen to 52.6% in case of resistant microorganisms [2]. The rate can be reduced to only 18% when these microorganisms are identified and properly treated [19]. Maheshwari et al [2] reported that supracondylar amputation was performed on 14.2% of his cases, whereas only on 5.7% of his patients arthrodesis was the final operation. Our results show that infection was controlled in 75% of our patients with a knee arthrodesis done with a cemented modular nail and no more re-operations were needed. In our series, just one case of amputation was performed (5%). We agree with others authors [13, 20] that after a second TKA infection due to high virulence microorganisms or after multiple attempts of failed revision arthroplasty, knee arthrodesis should be the therapeutic choice in most of the cases or at least in those cases with low functional demanding patients in order to avoid a possible supracondylar amputation.

The three most frequent surgical techniques used to achieved knee arthrodesis after failed TKA are internal plate fixation, intramedullary rod fixation and external fixation [4]. Subsequent conversion of a knee arthrodesis to a total knee arthroplasty is not advisable, as almost of the reimplanted arthroplasties fail [21, 22].

Internal plate fixation is rarely used to achieve knee fusion due to the requirement of a broad soft tissue exposure, long time weight-bearing and because of the incidence of pseudoarthrosis is high.

External fixation has been the method of choice to attained knee arthrodesis following chronic infected TKA [8, 9, 23-25]. Advantages of external fixation include the fact that produces proper bone compression, the surgical procedure can be performed in one operative stage, and no implants remain inside the body after the external fixator removal. These details presume less recurrent infection rate than other arthrodesis techniques. Problems related to this treatment are carrying the device for long periods of time, usually more than six months, the subsequent shortening of the limb, the pin site infection or the possibility of a fracture through the weakened bone [7]. Nowadays this alternative is used in chronic infected knees after arthrodesis with bad tolerance of the nail. [4]. Two of our patients (10% of cases) needed an external fixator (Illizarov method) to achieve a useful limb.

Intramedullary nail is actually the most widespread option to fuse the knee [4, 20, 26-29]. Rate of fusion near 100% has been well documented in literature, as well as the satisfactory results in case of persistent infection that rarely forces the surgeon to take out the nail [30]. Complications of intramedullary nail fixation include periprosthetic fracture, hardware-related pain, bone loosening and persistent infection. Arthrodesis performed with a nail should be done according to a two-staged protocol in order to reduce the incidence of reinfection. Two of our four cases (50%), which showed inadequate infection control, were treated in first instance through a one-stage surgery; this fact supports previous reports and remarks the requirement of two stage-surgery to get a free-infected arthrodesis [4,31,32].

The preference of achieving knee fusion with an external fixator or with the aid of an intramedullary rod should be based on surgeon's experience and on the review of the advantages and disadvantages of each techniques [7].

There are different models of knee nails used to achieve arthrodesis. In the beginning long Küntscher nail was introduced through the great trochanter after debridement of the infected joint [33, 34]. This double approach is rarely used nowadays, and is reserved to failures of previous arthrodesis, fractures of the tibia or femur or cases of bone loosening that requires extended fixation [35, 36]. One patient (5%) of our series needed this procedure.

Modular nail can be inserted through the knee and it is at the present time the most frequent surgical technique to achieve a knee fusion; it shows fusion rates of nearly 95% of cases [37-39]. Modular nails could be cemented or uncemented but there is no literature that compares results of these models. When an uncemented nail is used, maximum bone contact is extremely important in order to get knee arthrodesis and usually autologous bone graft is required. After using an uncemented device shortening of the limb is frequent, as occurs with external fixators. Fractures around the tip of the rod or the locked screws are possible [40], as well as loosening of the implant. Few reports and small number of cases with the use of cemented nails have been published, so hardly any conclusions about this procedure can be obtained [10, 11]. The technique of cementing the nail could avoid shortening of the limb, compensate bone loss and provide an artificial joint fusion without employing bone graft. Fractures around the nail are probably less frequent than in uncemented nails, but when cemented nails must be removed surgery is quite tougher and bone loss bone could be a problem for the revision surgeries. Neuerburg et al [11] have published a review with the same number of cases than us, with similar results and conclusions, advising of clinical and radiological follow-up to allow appropriate surgery in case of loosening.

5. Conclusion

Recurrent infection after a previously exchange arthroplasty for chronic infected TKA is a challenging problem. This devastating complication is associated to infection due to high virulence resistant microorganisms, poor soft tissue coverage and a high number of previous surgeries. When this complication occurs, surgeons must always have in mind the possibility of an above knee amputation as a final result if we insist on revising to a knee arthroplasty. In order to avoid this terrible result, knee arthrodesis, preferably in two-stages, could be an option to achieve a useful and stable painless limb. Among the different alternatives to obtain knee arthrodesis, we believe that the best procedure is inserting a cemented modular nail through the knee, which provides a strong fixation, has a low rate of reinfection and allows to restore the length of the limb though significant bone loss due to previous surgeries.

Author details

Pablo Renovell, Antonio Silvestre and Oscar Vaamonde

Orthopaedic Department. Hospital Clínico of Valencia, Spain

References

[1] Blom, A. W, Brown, J, Taylor, A. H, Pattison, G, Whitehouse, S, & Bannister, G. C. Infection after total knee arthroplasty. J Bone Joint Surg Br. (2004). Jul;, 86(5), 688-91.

[2] Maheshwari, A. V, Gioe, T. J, Kalore, N. V, & Cheng, E. Y. Reinfection after prior staged reimplantation for septic total knee arthroplasty: is salvage still possible? J Arthroplasty. (2010). Sep; 25(6 Suppl): , 92-7.

[3] Morrey, B. F, Westholm, F, Schoifet, S, Rand, J. A, & Bryan, R. S. Long-term results of various treatment options for infected total knee arthroplasty. Clin Orthop Relat Res. (1989). Nov;(248): 120-8.

[4] Conway, J. D, Mont, M. A, & Bezwada, H. P. Arthrodesis of the knee. J Bone Joint Surg Am. (2004). Apr;A(4):835-48., 86.

[5] Wang, C. J, Huang, T. W, Wang, J. W, & Chen, H. S. The often poor clinical outcome of infected total knee arthroplasty. J Arthroplasty. (2002). Aug; , 17(5), 608-14.

[6] Husted, H. Toftgaard Jensen T. Clinical outcome after treatment of infected primary total knee arthroplasty. Acta Orthop Belg. (2002). , 68, 500-7.

[7] Mabry, T. M, Jacofsky, D. J, Haidukewych, G. J, & Hanssen, A. Comparison of intra-medullary nailing and external fixation knee arthrodesis for the infected knee replacement. Clin Orthop Relat Res. (2007). Nov; , 464, 11-5.

[8] Oostenbroek, H. J, & Van Roermund, P. M. Arthrodesis of the knee after an infected arthroplasty using the Ilizarov method. J Bone Joint Surg Br. (2001). Jan;, 83(1), 50-4.

[9] Manzotti, A, Pullen, C, Guerreschi, F, & Catagni, M. A. The Ilizarov method for failed knee arthrodesis following septic TKR. Knee. (2001). Jun;, 8(2), 135-8.

[10] Rao, M. C, Richards, O, Meyer, C, & Jones, R. S. Knee stabilisation following infected knee arthroplasty with bone loss and extensor mechanism impairment using a modular cemented nail. Knee. (2009). Dec; , 16(6), 489-93.

[11] Neuerburg, C, Bieger, R, Jung, S, Kappe, T, Reichel, H, & Decking, R. Bridging knee arthrodesis for limb salvage using an intramedullary cemented nail: a retrospective outcome analysis of a case series. Arch Orthop Trauma Surg. (2012). May 13.

[12] Dawson, J, Fitzpatrick, R, Murray, D, & Carr, A. Questionnarie on the perceptions of patients about total knee replacement. J Bone Joint Surg (Br) (1998). B: 63-9., 80.

[13] Klinger, H. M, Spahn, G, Schultz, W, & Baums, M. H. Arthrodesis of the knee after failed infected total knee arthroplasty. Knee Surg Sports Traumatol Arthrosc. (2006). May;, 14(5), 447-53.

[14] Sierra, R. J, Trousdale, R. T, & Pagnano, M. W. Above-the-knee amputation after a total knee replacement: prevalence, etiology, and functional outcome. J Bone Joint Surg Am. (2003). Jun; A(6):1000-4., 85.

[15] Fedorka, C. J, Chen, A. F, Mcgarry, W. M, & Parvizi, J. Klatt BA Functional ability after above-the-knee amputation for infected total knee arthroplasty. Clin Orthop Relat Res. (2011). Apr; , 469(4), 1024-32.

[16] Falahee, M. H, Matthews, L. S, & Kaufer, H. Resection arthroplasty as a salvage procedure for a knee with infection after a total arthroplasty. J Bone Joint Surg Am. (1987). , 69, 1013-21.

[17] Barrack, R. L, Engh, G, Rorabeck, C, et al. Patient satisfaction and outcome after septic versus aseptic revision total knee arthroplasty. J Arthroplasty 15:990, (2000).

[18] Benson, E. R, Resine, S. T, & Lewis, C. G. Functional outcome of arthrodesis for failed total knee arthroplasty. Orthopedics. (1998). , 21, 875-9.

[19] Kilgus, D. J, Howe, D. J, & Strang, A. Results of periprosthetic hip and knee infections caused by resistant bacteria. Clin Orthop Relat Res. (2002). Nov;(404):116-24.

[20] Wiedel, J. D. Salvage of infected total knee fusion: the last option. Clin Orthop Relat Res. (2002). Nov;(404):139-42.

[21] Naranja RJ JrLotke PA, Pagnano MW, Hanssen AD. Total knee arthroplasty in a previously ankylosed or arthrodesed knee. Clin Orthop. (1996). , 331, 234-7.

[22] Clemens, D, Lereim, P, & Holm, I. Reikerås O Conversion of knee fusion to total arthroplasty: complications in 8 patients. Acta Orthop. (2005). Jun;, 76(3), 370-4.

[23] Phillips, H. T, & Mears, D. C. Knee fusion with external skeletal fixation after an infected hinge prosthesis: a case report. Clin Orthop Relat Res. (1980). Sep;(151):147-52.

[24] Garberina, M. J, Fitch, R. D, Hoffmann, E. D, Hardaker, W. T, Vail, T. P, & Scully, S. P. Knee arthrodesis with circular external fixation. Clin Orthop Relat Res. (2001). Jan;(382): 168-78.

[25] Vanryn, J. S, & Verebelyi, D. M. One-stage débridement and knee fusion for infected total knee arthroplasty using the hybrid frame. J Arthroplasty. (2002). Jan;, 17(1), 129-34.

[26] Wilde, A. H, & Stearns, K. L. Intramedullary fixation for arthrodesis of the knee after infected total knee arthroplasty. Clin Orthop Relat Res. (1989). Nov;(248):87-92.

[27] Gore, D. R, & Gassner, K. Use of an intramedullary rod in knee arthrodesis following failed total knee arthroplasty. J Knee Surg. (2003). Jul;, 16(3), 165-7.

[28] MacDonald JHAgarwal S, Lorei MP, Johanson NA, Freiberg AA. Knee arthrodesis. J Am Acad Orthop Surg. (2006). Mar;, 14(3), 154-63.

[29] Talmo, C. T, Bono, J. V, Figgie, M. P, Sculco, T. P, Laskin, R. S, & Windsor, R. E. Intramedullary arthrodesis of the knee in the treatment of sepsis after TKR. HSS J. (2007). Feb;, 3(1), 83-8.

[30] Schoifet, S. D, & Morrey, B. Persistent infection after successful arthrodesis for infected total knee arthroplasty. A report of two cases. J Arthroplasty. (1990). Sep;, 5(3), 277-9.

[31] Knutson, K, Hovelius, L, Lindstrand, A, & Lidgren, L. Arthrodesis after failed knee arthroplasty. Clin Orthop. (1984).

[32] Elligsen, D. E. Rand, JA Intramedullary arthrodesis of the knee after failed total knee arthroplasty. J Bone Joint Surg (1994). A:870-877., 76.

[33] Mazet R JrUrist MR. Arthrodesis of the knee with intramedullary nail fixation. Clin Orthop. (1960). , 18, 43-53.

[34] Knutson, K, & Lidgren, L. Arthrodesis after infected knee arthroplasty using an intramedullary nail. Reports of four cases. Arch Orthop Trauma Surg. (1982). , 100(1), 49-53.

[35] Jorgensen, P. S, & Torholm, C. Arthrodesis after infected knee arthroplasty using long arthrodesis nail. A report of five cases. Am J Knee Surg. (1995). , 8, 110-3.

[36] Bargiotas, K, Wohlrab, D, Sewecke, J. J, Lavinge, G, Demeo, P. J, & Sotereanos, N. G. Arthrodesis of the knee with a long intramedullary nail following the failure of a total knee arthroplasty as the result of infection. Surgical technique. J Bone Joint Surg Am. (2007). Mar;89 Suppl 2 Pt., 1, 103-10.

[37] Waldman, B. J, Mont, M. A, Payman, K. R, Freiberg, A. A, Windsor, R. E, Sculco, T. P, & Hungerford, D. S. Infected total knee arthroplasty treated with arthrodesis using a modular nail. Clin Orthop. (1999). , 367, 230-7.

[38] Mcqueen, D. A, Cooke, F. W, & Hahn, D. L. Knee arthrodesis with the Wichita Fusion Nail: an outcome comparison. Clin Orthop Relat Res. (2006). May;, 446, 132-9.

[39] Iacono, F, & Bruni, D. Lo Presti M, Raspugli G, Bondi A, Sharma B, Marcacci M. Knee arthrodesis with a press-fit modular intramedullary nail without bone-on-bone fusion after an infected revision TKA. Knee. (2012). Oct;Epub 2012 Feb 15., 19(5), 555-9.

[40] Hinarejos, P, Ginés, A, Monllau, J. C, Puig, L, & Cáceres, E. Fractures above and below a modular nail for knee arthrodesis. A case report. Knee. (2005). Jun;, 12(3), 231-3.

Alternatives to Arthroplasty

Proximal Interphalangeal Joint Arthrodesis with Tendon Transfer of the Flexor Digitorum Brevis

Ricardo Becerro de Bengoa Vallejo,
Marta Elena Losa Iglesias and
Miguel Fuentes Rodriguez

Additional information is available at the end of the chapter

1. Introduction

Hammer toe is a deformity characterized by dorsiflexion of the metatarsophalangeal (MTP) joint, plantarflexion of the proximal interphalangeal (PIP) joint, and dorsiflexion of the distal interphalangeal (DIP) joint. Claw toe is a similar deformity characterized by dorsiflexion of the MTP and plantarflexion of the PIP and DIP joints. These terms are often used interchangeably because both deformities involve the MTP joint. [1]

The causes of dorsiflexion of the metatarso- and interphalangeal joint have been described by various authors. [3], [4], [5], [6] Sandeman [2] reported that when the proximal phalanx is in the dorsal position at the expense of MTP dorsiflexion, the axis of the intrinsic musculature shifts. This causes a loss of competence of the intrinsic musculature of the foot, and the proximal phalanx can no longer be maintained in a plantar position. In the presence of concurrent flexor digitorum longus (FDL) contraction, the intrinsic musculature loses its ability to plantarflex the MTP joint. In a closed kinetic chain, this causes pathologic dorsiflexion of the MTP joint and places the proximal phalanx in a dorsal position. The result is claw or hammer deformity of the involved digits. Surgical correction of claw and hammer toe deformities utilize the action of the FDL tendon transferred to transform the deforming forces into corrective forces.

Correction of this flexible digital deformity by means of tendinous transposition of the flexor musculature to the extensor region of the toes has been described. [7], [8], [9], [10], [11], [12], [13] In each instance two cutaneous incisions have been utilized, one dorsal and another plantar. Only Barbari and Brevig [9] have described FDL tendon transfer to the dorsum of the extensor digitorum longus (EDL) tendon through a single incision approach. In this approach the dorso-lateral incision over the MTP joint extends about 3 cm distally from the neck of the metatarsal bone when there is only a single involved digit. When the procedure is undertaken in multiple digits, a transverse incision at the level of the digit crease is performed and the FDL tendon is sutured end-to-side to the EDL tendon. The authors stated that care must be taken to avoid injuring the neurovascular axes which are retracted laterally. The authors also advocated, when indicated, performing plantar capsulotomies for the DIP and PIP joints as described by Pyper [12] and Taylor. [13] The additional incision, however, increases the risk for injuring the principal plantar vessels of the involved digits..

Thus far, it has been recommended that correction of claw and hammer toe deformities be performed by transferring the FDL tendon to the dorsum of the proximal phalanx. Transposition of the FDL tendon via the dorsal approach through a unique longitudinal dorsal cutaneous incision without performing plantar incisions for capsulotomies of the DIP and PIP joints has not been previously described. To determine the feasibility of transferring the FDL tendon as an approach to correct claw and hammer toe deformities with this approach, it is necessary to determine whether these fascicles are long enough to transpose to the plantar aspect of the EDL tendon in the dorsal area of the proximal phalanx, and directly to the dorsum of the proximal phalanx of the second and third toes. We hypothesized that the FDL tendon, when incised at the level of the PIP joint, has adequate anatomical length to be transferred to the dorsal aspect of the proximal phalanx via a single longitudinal dorsal cutaneous incision and it would not be necessary to perform plantar capsulotomies at the interphalangeal joints, thus decreasing the risk of injury to the principal plantar vessels of the digits.

2. Materials and methods

Sixty cadaveric foot specimens (Total N, 60; 30 right, 30 left) were used for study procedures, including fourteen fresh and forty-six embalmed specimens. Transfer of the FDL tendon to the dorsum of the proximal phalanx via dorsal approach was attempted in 120 toes (60 each second and third toes).

The surgical technique performed in this study was a modification of a previously described method to transfer the flexor digitorum brevis (FDB) tendon. [14] To perform the FDL transfer a central longitudinal incision was made on the dorsal aspect of the digit, preserving the medial and lateral vessels and nerves. The incision was along the dorsum of the proximal phalanx of the digit from the base to the PIP joint. Once the EDL tendon was exposed, it was tenomiced and released along with the transverse aponeurosis that shapes the digital extensor apparatus. Proximal phalanx arthroplasty and hood ligament and MTP joint release were then performed by means of a dorsal, medial, and lateral capsulotomy. Section of the collateral and suspensory ligaments was performed to reduce the fixed extension deformity of the MTP joint in the specimens with fixed claw or hammer toe deformities.

After arthroplasty of the proximal phalanx was completed the dorsal aspect of the distal tendon sheath of the FDL and FDB tendons was exposed (Fig. 1). The vincula from the plantar aspect of the proximal phalanx to the dorsal aspect of the FDL and FDB tendons were released to further expose the flexor tendon sheath (Fig. 2). The tendon sheath was then incised and split longitudinally to the base of the middle phalanx (Fig. 3A), and the medial and lateral hemi-tendons of the FDB were exposed dorsally to the FDL (Fig. 3B). Plantar exposure of the FDB tendon was performed by inserting a curved hemostat by means of a blunt technique to identify and isolate the medial and lateral fascicles (Fig. 4 A, B). If the hemitendons of the FDB were not split adequately to permit passage of the FDL tendon, the FDB was divided longitu-dinally and proximally using a #15 blade (Fig. 5). The lateral and medial FDB hemitendons were then retracted to expose the FDL tendon (Fig. 6). Using a curved hemostat the FDL was collected dorsally between the medial and lateral FDB hemitendons (Fig. 7). Using a mini-osteotome, the FDL tendon was released from the plantar aspect of the distal middle phalanx to maximize the available tendon length (Fig. 8). This technique maximizes the length of the free distal tendinous stump to facilitate transfer to the dorsal aspect of the proximal phalanx (Fig. 9). The free proximal end of the tendon was clamped for later transfer (Fig 10). Next, using a #15 blade, the long flexor was split longitudinally in two portions, lateral and medial, proximal to distal (Fig. 11). Both free proximal FDL tendons were exposed between the plantar aspect of the proximal phalanx and the dorsal aspect of the FDB tendons (Fig 12).

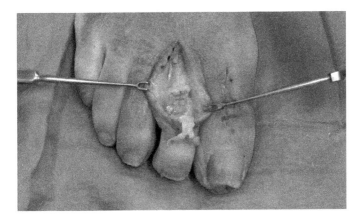

Figure 1. Dorsal aspect of the second digit after arthroplasty of the proximal phalanx and release of the metatarso-phalangeal joint. The base of the middle phalanx is exposed. The proximal phalanx with the head resected is shown, and plantarly is the digital segment of the distal tendon sheath of the flexor digitorum longus and brevis tendons.

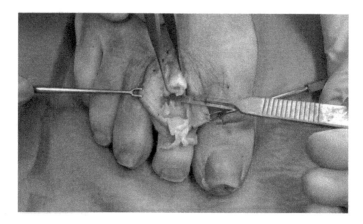

Figure 2. The plantar vincula are sectioned to release the flexor tendon sheath at the plantar aspect of the proximal phalanx of the second digit.

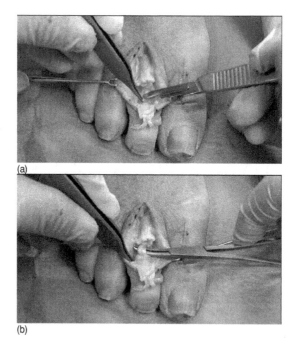

(a)

(b)

Figure 3. (a) The tendinous sheath is cut longitudinally, proximally and distally to the base of the middle phalanx. **(b)** The tendinous sheath is opened, and the flexor digitorum brevis hemitendons, lateral and medial, are exposed over the curved hemostat.

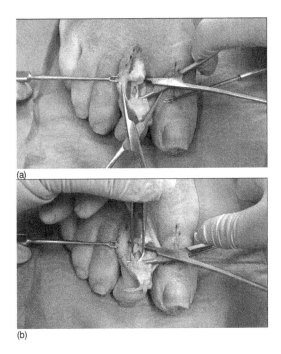

(a)

(b)

Figure 4. (a) The medial and lateral fascicles of the flexor digitorum brevis tendon are isolated using a curved hemostat. The flexor digitorum longus is localized plantarly. **(b)** Dorsal view of the hemitendons of flexor digitorum brevis with inadequate separation.

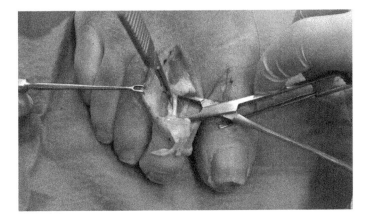

Figure 5. Flexor digitorum brevis is divided longitudinally and proximally using a blade #15 to permit passage of the flexor digitorum longus tendon.

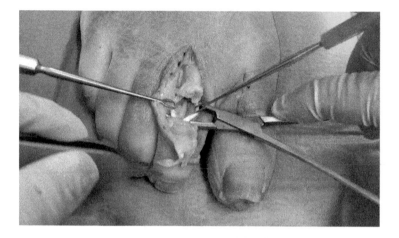

Figure 6. Medial and lateral hemitendon of the flexor digitorum brevis are retracted for plantar exposure of the flexor digitorum longus tendon.

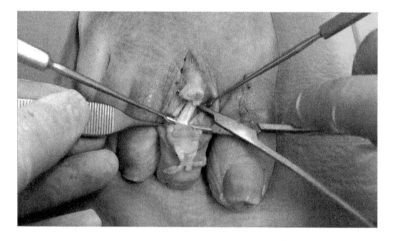

Figure 7. Using a curved hemostat and situating it plantar to the flexor digitorum longus is collocated dorsally between the medial and lateral hemitendons of flexor digitorum brevis.

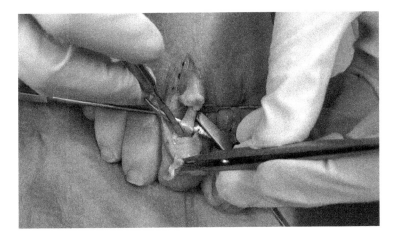

Figure 8. Using a mini-osteotome, the flexor digitorum longus tendon is released from the plantar aspect of the middle phalanx distally to obtain more tendon to facilitate the transfer.

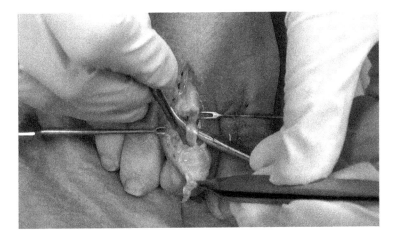

Figure 9. Flexor digitorum longus tendon is cut through its insertion point as distally as possible to the middle phalanx to maximize the length of the free distal tendinous stump.

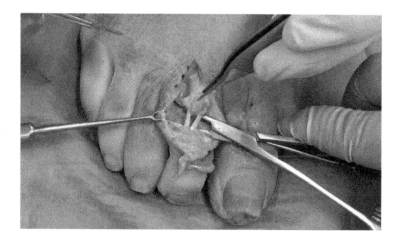

Figure 10. The stump of the proximal flexor digitorum longus tendon is clamped.

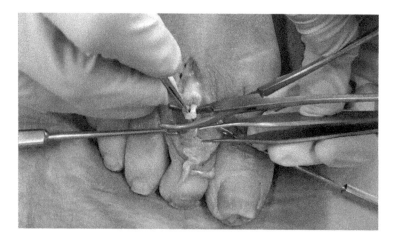

Figure 11. The long flexor is split longitudinally using a #15 blade.

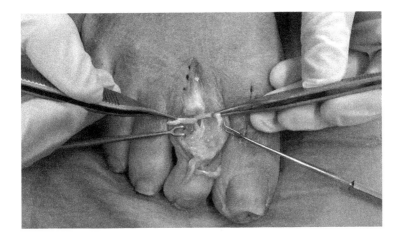

Figure 12. The flexor digitorum longus tendon has been split longitudinally in two portions, lateral and medial.

Once the medial and lateral fascicles of the FDL tendon had been clamped they were trans-ferred to the dorsal aspect of the medial and lateral proximal phalanx, respectively. During this procedure the length of the split tendinous fascicles of the FDL tendon were evaluated to ascertain whether the length was sufficient to permit transposition over the dorsal proximal phalanx. If the length was not adequate, a major incision was made in the proximal flexor tendon sheath. The medial and lateral FDL tendon stumps were sutured to itself in the dorsum of the proximal phalanx (Fig. 13 A,B,C,D).

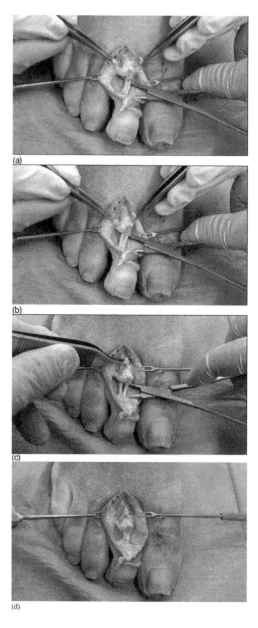

(a)

(b)

(c)

(d)

Figure 13. (a and b) The medial and lateral fascicles of the flexor digitorum longus tendon are transferred to the dorsal area of the proximal phalanx. The hemostat is showing the flexor digitorum brevis hemitendons. **(c)** Dorsal view of the medial and lateral stumps of the flexor digitorum longus tendon transferred to the medial and lateral aspects of the proximal phalanx, respectively, and clamped with a pick up. The hemostat is showing the flexor digitorum brevis hemitendons intact. **(d)** Dorsal view of the flexor digitorum longus transferred to the dorsal aspect of the proximal phalanx

The toe was pinned using a double-pointed 0.54-mm Kirschner wire in a retrograde manner driven antegrade from the PIP joint, out the tip of the toe, and then retrograde into the proximal phalanx and the metatarsal head. The EDL stumps were sutured over the transferred FDL tendon (Fig. 14), and cutaneous suturing was performed in a usual manner.

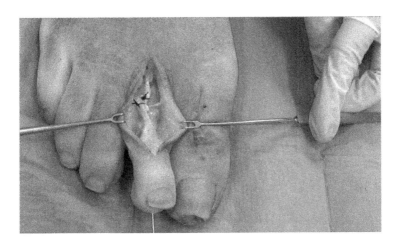

Figure 14. The extensor digitorum longus tendon stumps are sutured over the transferred flexor digitorum longus tendon.

3. Results

The FDL tendon transfer by the unique longitudinal dorsal approach attempted on 120 cadaveric toes (60 second toes and 30 third toes) was successful in 100% of the cases.

4. Discussion

The results of this study indicate that transfer of the FDL tendinous fascicles between the FDB hemitendons can be performed on second and third digits via a unique dorsal incision. Success of the procedure is predicated, in part, on an adequate longitudinal incision of the flexor tendon sheath that permits exposure and separation of the FDB hemitendons. We believe the indications for FDL tendon transfer between FDB hemitendons are the same as those for the FDL tendon transfer that other authors [28]- [36] are using for the correction of sagittal plane lesser MTP joint instability and loss of digital purchase. We do not, however, advocate this approach when the fifth digit is involved. In the current investigation, the FDB tendon was absent in 3 cases (7%), thus the dorsal approach was not possible. Any hammer toe or claw toe deformity that is accompanied by a semi-rigid or rigid MTP joint requires accompanying correction. This correction may be accomplished via PIP joint fusion or FDL tendon transfer, which moves the lever arm to the MTP joint and holds the proximal phalanx in a plantarflexed position.

Based on the results of this investigation, we believe the surgical technique for FDL tendon transfer should utilize a dorsal approach to minimize the risk of compromising the principal blood supply to the involved digits. Chen et al [37] evaluated the vasculature of 20 foot specimens focusing on the second, third, and fourth toes. Findings from the study suggest that plantar circulation is predominant in the second, third, and fourth toes, while dorsal circulation predominated in the first digit. Chen et al [37] further stated that the plantar digital arteries of the lesser toes provide the predominant arterial supply of the PIP joints through a system of transverse and longitudinal arches. Thus, when a claw or hammer toe deformity correction is performed via FDL tendon transfer through a two-incision plantar approach, a decision must be made regarding whether to continue or discontinue surgery when there is a risk of vascular compromise to the digit due to two incisions. Emphasizing the potential deleterious consequences of multiple incisions, Coughlin [18] recommended that it is far better to offer a 2-stage repair of the deformity than to incur a vascular insult with excessive surgery on a digit.

Surgical correction of hammer and claw toe deformity has been described extensively. Transposition of the flexor tendon to the extensor musculature through a dorso-lateral cut, with FDL tendon transfer to the dorso-lateral area of the proximal phalanx, was originally performed by Girdlestone in 1947 and developed by Taylor. [13] In his study, Taylor included 68 patients with claw or hammer toe deformity treated with this technique and associated procedures, such as dorsal capsulotomy of the MTP joint. Taylor also performed plantar capsulotomy of the interphalangeal joints and stabilization of the proximal phalanx using an external splint. Several modifications of the procedure have subsequently been reported. In 1970, Sgarlato [16] reported 53 cases of FDL tendon transfer through 3 skin incisions. Pyper [12] performed the technique described by Taylor [13] on 45 feet in 23 patients. To correct the digital deformity, he combined it with lengthening of the EDL tendon and dorsal capsulotomy of the MTP joint. Subsequently, Parrish [11] modified this technique by detaching the FDL tendon and dividing the proximal tendinous stump longitudinally and repositioning its medial and lateral aspects in the extensor area. He performed FDL and FDB tendon transfer on the first 5 patients in his series but not on the remaining 18 patients, stating that "the FDB tendon had a smaller calibre and its length was insufficient for the transposition." [11]

Marcinko et al [17] described the FDL tendon transfer using two incisions in the toe, one plantar and another dorsal. Barbari and Brevig [9] performed 39 FDL transpositions to the extensor area in 31 patients; 11 of the 39 procedures were performed in accordance with the technique of Taylor, [13] with the remaining 28 following the modified technique described by Parrish. [11] The approach was through a dorso-lateral incision over the MTP joint extending approximately 3 cm distally from the neck of the metatarsal bone. Dissection was then performed on each side of the proximal phalanx. The sheath of the flexor tendons was located, and the long flexor was then isolated, drawn out using a blunt hook, and divided near its distal insertion. It was then sutured end to end to the extensor tendon.

Coughlin [18], [19] performed an FDL tendon transfer by first making a transverse incision at the MTP joint, and then a second incision at the dorsal aspect of the digit. Kuwada [20] performed 81 procedures to transfer the FDL tendon via a dorsolateral incision along the digit beginning proximally at the MTP joint and extending distally to least the proximal PIP joint. Thompson and Deland [21] performed transfer of the FDL tendon in 13 digits following the indications of Coughlin [18] via the plantar and dorsal approach. Gazdag and Cracchiolo [22] in 11 feet performed an isolating tendon transfer of the FDL through the 2-cm longitudinal midline incision on the plantar side of the base of the proximal phalanx and performed another dorsal incision at the base of the proximal phalanx. Recently, Boyer and DeOrio [23] treated 70 toes with fixed or flexible hammer toes with a flexor-to-extensor tendon transfer making a longitudinal incision on the plantar aspect of the proximal phalanx and at the dorsal aspect of the toe.

The literature up to now reveals no attempts to discover why Parrish [11] found FDB tendon transfer to be a non-viable option. His findings, however, have been accepted by the scientific community without confirmation or challenge. Furthermore, many of the authors cited, except Barbari and Brevig, [9] performed the double plantar and dorsal incision approach as described by Girdlestone in 1947. [13]

In a cadaveric study we found [14] that it is possible to correct flexible claw and hammer toe deformity by transposing the FDB tendon to the extensor, or dorsal, area of the base of the proximal phalanx. This is a modification of the procedure used by Parrish [11] using a plantar and dorsal incision approach of the digit. We sought to transfer the FDB tendon to the dorsal aspect of the proximal phalanx via the dorsal approach through a unique incision, as described by Barbari and Brevig. [9]A search of the indexed literature found no previous reports of this procedure.

It is possible anatomical variations in the insertion of the FDB tendon may prohibit the popularity of this transfer approach. Three variations have been described: 1) absence of the tendon; 2) absence of the lateral and medial tendinous fascicles but presence of a single tendon running parallel to the FDL tendon; and 3) fusion of the FDB tendon to the FDL tendon. [24]-[27] LeDouble [24] and Nathan and Gloobe [25] found the FDB tendon to be absent in the fifth toe in 21.5% of cases. Testut [27] found the FDB tendon to be absent in the fourth and fifth toes in 3% of the dissections performed. In two separate studies [26], [27] Testut found that the FDB medial and lateral fascicles are not divided. Rather, the fascicles run parallel to the FDL tendon before inserting into a side of the intermediate phalanx of the fifth or fourth toe in 5% of patients. Although Testut [26], [27] did not specify individual percentages for variability in attachment for each of these digits, he established that the FDB tendon of the fifth toe is fused to the FDL tendon in 2% of cases. Thus, the anatomical variations found occur more frequently in the FDB tendon insertion of the fifth toe.

Anomalies or variations in the insertion of the FDB tendon in the third and second toes have not, however, been described. We reported [14] on transposition of the FDB tendon via the plantar approach in 180 digits of cadaveric feet, including 45 second digits, 45 third digits, 45 fourth digits, and 45 fifth digits. We found no cases of variation in the insertion of the FDB tendon in the second, third, or fourth digits, and the FDB tendon was present in all 45 cases. There was variability in FDB tendon presentation in the fifth digit, including FDB tendon absence in 3 of 45 digits (7%), which is a recognized anatomical variation. Thus, we performed the dorsal FDL tendon transfer via the dorsal approach between the FDB hemitendons in only the second and third digits.

Another potential factor prohibiting the tendon transfer approach described in this study may be inadequate space for FDL passage through the FDB hemitendons. After arthroplasty the tendon sheath is exposed and opened longitudinally, and the hemitendons of the FDB are identified just over the FDL tendon. Once the hemitendons are identified they are carefully separated (Fig. 4). If there is not adequate room for FDL passage, the FDB hemitendons must be incised longitudinally (Fig. 5). We believe this additional surgical step is the primary challenge associated with this technique, and may potentially explain why this technique has not previously been described.

Available FDL tendon length may also impact the surgical approach. Once the FDL tendon is detached distally from the distal phalange, it must be long enough to be transposed to the dorsal aspect of the proximal phalanx. When the MTP joint is rigidly dorsiflexed, it is necessary to perform a dorsal capsulotomy and MTP joint release as described by Barbari and Brevig, [9] thus relocating the proximal phalanx to its anatomical position. With this approach there is no need for plantar capsulotomies of the interphalangeal joints.

If there is difficulty in transferring the distal stumps of the longitudinally split FDL tendon to the dorsal aspect of the proximal phalanx of any digit, the clinician must cut the proximal flexor tendon sheath longitudinally for better FDL tendon exposure. We were able to transfer the FDL tendon via dorsal approach between the FDB hemitendons in 100% of second and third digits via a unique single longitudinal incision. We did find it difficult, however, to transfer the FDL "around" the lateral aspects of the FDB hemitendons. This transfer was unsuccessful in 83 (69,16%; N = 120) digits, including 45 (37,5%) second digits and 38 (31,66%) of the third digits. We believe this was a consequence of inadequate proximal tendon sheath dissection. When attempting transfer of the split FDL tendon lateral to the FDB hemitendons, it is difficult to obtain adequate proximal exposure secondary to the depth of the anatomical structures. A mini-osteotome may be used to release the FDL tendon from the plantar aspect of the distal middle phalanx to obtain more tendon and facilitate the transfer.

While passing the split FDL tendons between the hemitendons of the FDB is necessary to cut the flexor tendon sheath.

We also encountered difficulty in transposing the FDL tendon as a consequence of the transverse aponeurotic fibers originating from the EDL tendon. These fibers surround the MTP joint capsule and join in the plantar area with the glenoid plate, the deep MTP ligament, and the sheath of the flexor tendons to insert distally into the plantar base of the proximal phalanx. These aponeurotic fibers and the sheath of the flexor tendons must be cut to allow the split FDL tendon to be repositioned and sutured to the dorsal aspect of the proximal phalanx.

A final challenge associated with this novel surgical approach is ankle positioning while suturing FDL tendon stumps. If the ankle is in plantarflexion the tendon has adequate length to permit suturing to the dorsal aspect of the proximal phalanx without difficulty. When the patient is weight-bearing or walking, however, the ankle is in dorsiflexion, which shortens the FDL tendon and forces the MTP joint into plantarflexion. The FDL tendon should therefore be sutured in its anatomical position to avoid inappropriate flexion or extension positioning of any involved joint.

5. Conclusions

Transfer of the FDL tendon to the dorsum of the proximal phalanx can be performed for the correction of claw and hammer toe deformities in the second and third digits. The meticulous longitudinal incision of the flexor tendon sheath to expose the FDB tendon and its longitudinal incision are essential to the success of the procedure. Furthermore, this approach preserves the integrity of the primary plantar blood supply to the digits of interest.

Author details

Ricardo Becerro de Bengoa Vallejo[1*], Marta Elena Losa Iglesias[2] and Miguel Fuentes Rodriguez[1]

*Address all correspondence to: ibebeva@enf.ucm.es

1 Escuela Universitaria de Enfermería, Fisioterapia y Podología, Universidad Complutense de Madrid, Madrid, Spain

2 Facultad de Ciencias de la Salud, Universidad Rey Juan Carlos, Madrid, Spain

References

[1] Coughlin, M. J. Lesser-toe abnormalities. J Bone Joint Surg Am (2002). , 84, 1446-1469.

[2] Sandeman, J. C. The role of soft tissue correction of claw toes. Br J Clin Pract (1967). , 21, 489-93.

[3] Coughlin, M. J, & Mann, R. A. Lesser Toe Deformities. In: MJ Coughlin, RA Mann Surgery of the Foot and Ankle, 7th ed. Mosby, St Louis; (1999). , 328.

[4] Richardson, E. G. Lesser Toe Abnormalities. In: AH Crenshaw. Campbell's Operative Orthopaedics, 8th ed. Mosby-Year Book, St Louis; (1992). , 99.

[5]   Scheck, M. Etiology of acquired hammertoe deformity. Clin Orthop. (1977). , 123, 63-9.

[6]   Engle, E. T, & Morton, D. J. Notes on foot disorders among natives of the Belgian Congo. J Bone Joint Surg. (1931).

[7]   Lutter, L. D. Toe Deformities. In: *Atlas of Adult Foot and Ankle Surgery,* Mosby-Year Book, St Louis; (1997). , 74.

[8]   Cyphers, S. M, & Feiwell, E. Review of the Girdlestone-Taylor procedure for claw-toes in myelodysplasia. Foot Ankle. (1988). , 8, 229-33.

[9]   Barbari, S. G, & Brevig, K. Correction of clawtoes by the Girdlestone-Taylor flexor-extensor transfer procedure. Foot Ankle. (1984). , 5, 67-73.

[10] Newman, R. J, & Fitton, J. M. An evaluation of operative procedures in the treatment of hammertoe. Acta Orthop Scand. (1979). , 50, 709-12.

[11] Parrish TF: Dynamic correction of clawtoesOrthop Clin North Am. (1973). , 4, 97-102.

[12] Pyper, J. B. The flexor-extensor transplant operation for claw toes. J Bone Joint Surg Br. (1958). , 40, 528-33.

[13] Taylor, R. G. The treatment of claw toes by multiple transfers of flexor into extensor tendons. J Bone Joint Surg Br. (1951). , 33, 539-42.

[14] Becerro de Bengoa Vallejo RViejo Tirado F, Prados Frutos JC, Losa Iglesias ME, Jules KT. Transfer of the flexor digitorum brevis tendon. JAPMA. (2008). , 98, 27-35.

[15] Sarrafian, S. K. *Anatomy of the Foot and Ankle.* JB Lippincott, Philadelphia, (1983). , 243.

[16] Sgarlato, T. E. Transplantation of the flexor digitorum longus muscle tendon in ham-mertoes. JAPA. (1970). , 60, 383-8.

[17] Marcinko, D. E, Lazerson, A, Dollard, M. D, et al. Flexor digitorum longus tendon transfer: a simplified technique. JAPA. (1984). , 74, 380-5.

[18] Coughlin, M. J. Crossover second toe deformity. Foot Ankle. (1987). , 8, 29-39.

[19] Coughlin, M. J. Subluxation and dislocation of the second metatarsophalangeal joint. Orthop Clin North Am. (1989). , 20, 535-51.

[20] Kuwada, G. T. A retrospective analysis of modification of the flexor tendon transfer for correction of hammer toe. J Foot Surg. (1988). , 27, 57-9.

[21] Thompson, F. M, & Deland, J. T. Flexor tendon transfer for metatarsophalangeal in-stability of the second toe. Foot Ankle. (1993). , 14, 385-8.

[22] Gazdag, A, & Cracchiolo, A. Surgical treatment of patients with painful instability of the second metatarsophalangeal joint. Foot Ankle Int. (1998). , 19, 137-43.

[23] Boyer, M. L, & Deorio, J. K. Transfer of the flexor digitorum longus for the correction of lesser-toe deformities. Foot Ankle Int. (2007). , 28, 422-30.

[24] LeDouble AF *Traité des variations du systéme musculaire del l'homme et de leur signification au point de vue de l'anthropologie et zoologique,* Schleicher Fréres, Paris, (1897). , 2, 327.

[25] Nathan, H, & Gloobe, H. Flexor digitorum brevis: anatomical variations. Anat Anz. (1974). , 135, 295-301.

[26] Testut, L. *Les anomalies musculaires chez l'homme expliqueés par l'anatomie comparée: Leur importance en anthropologie.* Masson, Paris, (1884). , 588.

[27] Testut, L. *Les anomalies musculaires considérées du point de vue de la ligature des artéres.* Doin, Paris, (1892). , 38-40.

[28] Thompson, F. M, & Deland, J. T. Flexor tendon transfer for metatarsophalangeal instability of the second toe. Foot Ankle. (1993).

[29] Gazdag, A, & Cracchiolo, A. Surgical treatment of patients with painful instability of the second metatarsophalangeal joint. Foot Ankle Int. (1998).

[30] Coughlin, M. J. Second metatarsophalangeal joint instability in the athlete. Foot Ankle Int. (1993).

[31] Kuwada, G. T. A retrospective analysis of modification of the flexor tendon transfer for correction of hammertoe. J Foot Surg. (1988).

[32] Coughlin, M. J. Subluxation and dislocation of the second metatarsophalangeal joint. Orthop Clin North Am. (1989).

[33] Thompson, F. M, & Deland, J. T. Flexor tendon transfer for metatarsophalangeal instability of the second toe. Foot Ankle Int. (1993). , 14, 385-8.

[34] Mendocino, R. W, Statler, T. K, Saltrick, K. R, & Catanzariti, A. R. Predislocation syndrome: a review and analysis of eight patients. J Foot Ankle Surg. (2001). , 40, 214-24.

[35] Myerson, M. S, & Jung, H. G. The role of toe flexor-to-extensor transfer in correcting metatarsophalangeal joint instability of the second toe. Foot Ankle Int. (2005). , 29, 675-9.

[36] Bouché, R. T, & Heit, E. J. Combined plantar plate and hammertoe repair with flexor digitorum longus tendon transfer for chronic, severe sagittal plane instability of the lesser metatarsophalangeal joints: preliminary observations. J Foot Ankle Surg. (2008). , 47, 125-37.

[37] Chen, Y. G, Cook, P. A, Mcclinton, M. A, et al. Microarterial anatomy of the lesser toe proximal interphalangeal joints. J Hand Surg [Am]. (1998). , 23, 256-60.

[38] May JW JrChait LA, Cohen BE, O'Brien BM. Free neurovascular flap from the first web space of the foot in hand reconstruction. J Hand Surg. (1977). , 2, 387-93.

[39] Murakami T: On the position and course of the deep plantar arterieswith special reference to the so-called plantar metatarsal arteries. Okajimas Folia Anat Jpn. (1971). , 48, 295-322.

Permissions

The contributors of this book come from diverse backgrounds, making this book a truly international effort. This book will bring forth new frontiers with its revolutionizing research information and detailed analysis of the nascent developments around the world.

We would like to thank Plamen Kinov, MD, PhD, for lending his expertise to make the book truly unique. He has played a crucial role in the development of this book. Without his invaluable contribution this book wouldn't have been possible. He has made vital efforts to compile up to date information on the varied aspects of this subject to make this book a valuable addition to the collection of many professionals and students.

This book was conceptualized with the vision of imparting up-to-date information and advanced data in this field. To ensure the same, a matchless editorial board was set up. Every individual on the board went through rigorous rounds of assessment to prove their worth. After which they invested a large part of their time researching and compiling the most relevant data for our readers. Conferences and sessions were held from time to time between the editorial board and the contributing authors to present the data in the most comprehensible form. The editorial team has worked tirelessly to provide valuable and valid information to help people across the globe.

Every chapter published in this book has been scrutinized by our experts. Their significance has been extensively debated. The topics covered herein carry significant findings which will fuel the growth of the discipline. They may even be implemented as practical applications or may be referred to as a beginning point for another development. Chapters in this book were first published by InTech; hereby published with permission under the Creative Commons Attribution License or equivalent.

The editorial board has been involved in producing this book since its inception. They have spent rigorous hours researching and exploring the diverse topics which have resulted in the successful publishing of this book. They have passed on their knowledge of decades through this book. To expedite this challenging task, the publisher supported the team at every step. A small team of assistant editors was also appointed to further simplify the editing procedure and attain best results for the readers.

Our editorial team has been hand-picked from every corner of the world. Their multi-ethnicity adds dynamic inputs to the discussions which result in innovative outcomes. These outcomes are then further discussed with the researchers and contributors who give their valuable feedback and opinion regarding the same. The feedback is then collaborated with the researches and they are edited in a comprehensive manner to aid the understanding of the subject.

Apart from the editorial board, the designing team has also invested a significant amount of their time in understanding the subject and creating the most relevant covers. They scrutinized every image to scout for the most suitable representation of the subject and create an appropriate cover for the book.

The publishing team has been involved in this book since its early stages. They were actively engaged in every process, be it collecting the data, connecting with the contributors or procuring relevant information. The team has been an ardent support to the editorial, designing and production team. Their endless efforts to recruit the best for this project, has resulted in the accomplishment of this book. They are a veteran in the field of academics and their pool of knowledge is as vast as their experience in printing. Their expertise and guidance has proved useful at every step. Their uncompromising quality standards have made this book an exceptional effort. Their encouragement from time to time has been an inspiration for everyone.

The publisher and the editorial board hope that this book will prove to be a valuable piece of knowledge for researchers, students, practitioners and scholars across the globe.

List of Contributors

Asim Rajpura and Tim Board
Wrightington Hospital, Hall Lane, Appley Bridge, Wigan, Lancashire, UK

Pietro Melloni, Maite Veintemillas, Anna Marin and Rafael Valls
UDIAT Diagnostic Center, Corporació Sanitària i Universitària Parc Taulí, Sabadell, Spain

Vladan Stevanović
Institute for Orthopaedic Surgery Banjica, Belgrade, Serbia

Zoran Vukašinović , Zoran Baščarević and Duško Spasovski
Institute for Orthopaedic Surgery Banjica, Belgrade, Serbia Faculty of Medicine, University of Belgrade, Belgrade, Serbia

Branislav Starčević
Faculty of Medicine, University of Belgrade, Belgrade, Serbia Clinic for Orthopaedic Surgery and Traumatology, Clinical Center of Serbia, Belgrade, Serbia

Dragana Matanović
Faculty of Medicine, University of Belgrade, Belgrade, Serbia Clinic for Physical Therapy and Rehabilitation, Clinical Center of Serbia, Belgrade, Serbia

Raúl Lopez, Fernando Almeida, Pablo Renovell, Francisco Argüelles and Oscar Vaamonde
Clinic Hospital of Valencia, Spain

Antonio Silvestre
Clinic Hospital of Valencia, Spain Orthopedic Department, School of Medicine, University of Valencia, Spain

Nahum Rosenberg
Rambam – Health Care Campus, Laboratory of Musculoskeletal Research, Department of Orthopedic Surgery, Haifa, Israel

Maruan Haddad and Doron Norman
Rambam – Health Care Campus, Department of Orthopaedic Surgery. Haifa, Israel

Adrian J. Cassar Gheiti and Kevin J. Mulhall
Orthopedic Research and Innovation Foundation, Republic of Ireland

Michael Soudry
Department of Orthopaedic Surgery, Hillel Yaffe Medical Center, Hadera, Israel

Arnan Greental, Gabriel Nierenberg, Mazen Falah and Nahum Rosenberg
Rambam Health Care Campus, Dept. of Orthopedic Surgery. Haifa, Israel

Trisha Peel, Kirsty Buising, Michelle Dowsey and Peter Choong
University of Melbourne, St. Vincent's Hospital Melbourne, Australia

Manuel Villanueva-Martínez and Francisco Chana-Rodriguez
Hospital General Universitario Gregorio Marañón, Universidad Complutense de Madrid, Madrid, Spain

Antonio Ríos-Luna
Orthoindal Center, El Ejido, Almería University, Almería, Spain

Jose A. De Pedro
Hospital Universitario Salamanca, Salamanca University, Spain

Antonio Pérez-Caballer
Hospital Infanta Elena, Francisco de Vitoria University, Madrid, Spain

Pablo Renovell, Antonio Silvestre and Oscar Vaamonde
Orthopaedic Department, Hospital Clínico of Valencia, Spain

Ricardo Becerro de Bengoa Vallejo and Miguel Fuentes Rodriguez
Escuela Universitaria de Enfermería, Fisioterapia y Podología, Universidad Complutense de Madrid, Madrid, Spain

Marta Elena Losa Iglesias
Facultad de Ciencias de la Salud, Universidad Rey Juan Carlos, Madrid, Spain

Printed in the USA
CPSIA information can be obtained
at www.ICGtesting.com
JSHW011420221024
72173JS00004B/615

9 781632 410207